MISS BONNIE'S NURSES

Miss Bonnie's Nurses

The First Fifty Years of Nursing at
The University of North Carolina at Charlotte

Ann Mabe Newman, RN, PhD
Dona Harton Haney, RN, MSN

Suggested citation: Newman, Ann and Haney, Dona. Miss Bonnie's Nurses: The First Fifty
Years of Nursing at UNC Charlotte.
Charlotte: J. Murrey Atkins Library at UNC Charlotte, 2018.
doi: https://doi.org/10.5149/9781469647630_Newman

ISBN 978-1-4696-4761-6 (cloth: alk paper)
ISBN 978-1-4696-4762-3 (pbk: alk. paper)
ISBN 978-1-4696-4763-0 (ebook)

Published by the J. Murrey Atkins Library at UNC Charlotte

Distributed by the University of North Carolina Press
www.uncpress.org

CONTENTS

FOREWORD

Philip L. Dubois, Chancellor, UNC Charlotte

Consistently named by Gallup polls as "the most trusted profession," nursing is one of the most important, respected, and service-oriented careers one can choose. Who among us hasn't been affected by the kindness, efficiency, and compassion of a dedicated nurse?

Fifty years ago, UNC Charlotte celebrated the first graduating class of its new nursing program. And today, we celebrate the golden anniversary of what has become a gold standard of nursing education in our state, region, and nation.

In 1965, the proud legacy of nursing education at UNC Charlotte began with the determined efforts of three formidable women. Bonnie Cone, the founder of UNC Charlotte, recruited Edith Brocker from Duke University to become the first dean of nursing. Brocker then hired Elinor Caddell as the first faculty member, and a nursing program was born. During an era still dominated by men, this series of events is particularly significant.

Throughout my tenure at UNC Charlotte, first as provost and then as chancellor, I have been privileged to watch the evolution of our healthcare education programs as they have gone through many transitions to adapt to changing needs, technologies, and challenges within our society. As provost, I was particularly proud to have hired Dr. Sue Bishop, who served as dean of the College of Nursing and who led in the development of graduate specialty concentrations in the Community Health Nursing and Family Nurse Practitioner programs. Bishop's leadership in the expansion of our health education programming paved the way for an exciting period of growth.

In the following pages, you will read about the many heroes who built this program, who nurtured it during lean times, who envisioned what it could be, and who pushed boundaries to make that vision possible. Their stories inspire me, and I trust they will inspire you as well.

To those who set UNC Charlotte's nursing program into motion, to those who have dedicated their professional lives to educating future nurses here at UNC Charlotte, and to those who have studied here and gone on to provide excellent health care in their communities, I extend my sincere admiration and appreciation. Countless individuals for generations to come will benefit from your sacrificial dedication to this most noble and trusted profession.

Dee M. Baldwin, PhD, RN, FAAN,
Associate Dean and Director, School of Nursing, 2009–2017

I am pleased to contribute to the 50th anniversary of the School of Nursing to recognize the many accomplishments, successes, and milestones of the school, and to honor our faculty, staff, students, and alumni. The school is emerging as the premier nursing school in the region and is known for preparing nursing professionals who serve as leaders, experts, partners, and scholars to meet the healthcare needs of an ever-changing culturally diverse society. In these first 50 years, the school has enjoyed unprecedented growth, a strong reputation in the community, and a growing national prominence. Online graduate programs have risen in the rankings and have increased funding for undergraduate programs and access to students from underserved and underrepresented populations. The school has engaged in cutting-edge research in the area of vulnerable populations, and our faculty remain experts in addressing problems related to aging, health disparities, and chronic illness. Faculty have continued to lead in these existing and new areas of research, enabling the school to prepare graduates who can respond to changing and complex healthcare systems. The school has sought and recruited the very best from around the country to create an accomplished faculty and to attract top-notch students.

Our students, the reason for our existence, are bright and energetic. They are fundamental to our mission and vision. As we have enriched their experiences by embedding their education in evidence-based practice, nursing science, and cutting-edge research, they have taken every opportunity to use their talents in new, creative, and exciting ways to improve and strengthen the lives of the people and communities we serve. Our students are encouraged to take risks, remain true to our mission, and uphold our core values of excellence, integrity, scholarship, diversity, and collegiality. It is these values that have positioned and sustained us as a first-rate nursing school, one that has allowed us to dream big, strive for greatness, and work to become one of the leading schools in the region and beyond.

The school also prides itself on the partnerships that demonstrate, at the highest level, collaboration to provide innovative, individualized, and evidence-based nursing education. We have a notable record in working across disciplines and with others to create strong academic-community partnerships to enhance the knowledge and skill level of our students. In today's complex healthcare environment, nurses are required to be skilled professionals, critical thinkers, excellent communicators, and strong advocates for their patients and communities. These competencies, emanating from every aspect of our curricula, could not be achieved without the help of our partners. They help ensure that our students are educated and empowered to contribute in significant ways to shape health care and advance the science and practice of nursing.

I am so very proud to be a part of the school's strong history and legacy as the associate dean and director from 2009–17. Over the course of my eight-year tenure, the faculty, staff, and students worked together to continue to grow the school and our distinguished reputation of academic excellence. The school is a leader in both distance-based and simulation-based nursing education. Our laboratories continue to be a state-of-the-art teaching/learning environment, continually equipped with cutting-edge technology. During my tenure, I have seen growth and development in our offerings in the School of Nursing (SON) such as: a doubling of the enrollment in the RN-to-BSN program, the addition of an Early Entry option for the RN-to-MSN program, addition of the Adult Geriatric Acute Care Nurse Practitioner (AGACNP) to the MSN program, and creation of the school's first doctoral program—the dual UNC Charlotte/WCU Doctor of Nursing Practice (DNP).

The faculty are continually recognized for their contributions in preparing future nurses, practitioners, administrators, educators, and leaders in nursing as evidenced by personal recognition as well as the school's designation as a national Center of Excellence, awarded by the National League for Nursing. We also have a tremendous asset in our highly successful alumni and friends. I sought to strengthen the school's relationship with its alumni and encouraged them to play a more active role so that the school might draw on their knowledge, expertise, and experience. With this renewed connection, and with the support of the UNC Charlotte Alumni Association, the SON's alumni association (SONAC) was honored to become the first academic chapter on UNC Charlotte's campus, as opposed to an affinity-based alumni group. Each year, the SONAC offers an Annual Distinguished Alumni Lectureship Series that recognizes an alumnus who has made outstanding contributions to the school and the profession and will continue the tradition at the 50th anniversary of the School of Nursing on April 20, 2018.

The school has had an extraordinary first 50 years, and as UNC Charlotte continues to grow into a leading urban research university, the School of Nursing will grow its research mission, its community engagement, and its commitment to producing leaders, scholars, partners, and experts in health care. The next 50 years will build on the successes of the school's beginnings, focus on the challenges ahead, and respond to the needs of our citizens and communities. I am grateful to be a part of this ongoing history and great legacy, and look forward to what we will accomplish in the next 50 years. Here's wishing all the very best for the future and the next 50 years!

Growth and development is a process. And so it has been with this book. In 2004 for the 40th anniversary of the School of Nursing at UNC Charlotte, I was asked to compile a brief history to be used in a brochure. Fast forward to 2012. I retired and wrote a proposal for a book. "The college/school does not have a recorded history, and if one is not recorded now, much of the documentation may be lost forever," I wrote in the proposal. Maybe a slight exaggeration, but much of our history was contained in "The Box." A cardboard box of papers, newspaper clippings, pictures, and books from the days of Dean Edith Brocker in 1965 to the present (2017), the box had been lovingly moved to whatever space the College of Nursing (now School of Nursing in the College of Health and Human Services) occupied over the course of 50 years. At one point, we feared the box had been lost for good in the shuffle. Good detective work, a part of every nurse's repertoire of skills, found and saved our treasures.

In 2016, I again began compiling our history in more detail this time. A serendipitous conversation at a UNC Charlotte Nursing Alumni event moved the history from the box to the printed page. Dona Haney, RN, MSN, and I determined that, between the two of us, we were missing only four years of anecdotal history about the nursing program. Because of her previous experience in compiling and writing histories, I asked if she would be interested in joining me in writing *Miss Bonnie's Nurses: The First Fifty Years of Nursing at UNC Charlotte.* Little did I know what this dynamic detective would accomplish over the next year and a half. We collaborated on an outline, then Dona suggested focusing on the three early leaders in nursing education at UNC Charlotte. She researched and wrote brief biographies of each. Dona hunted down nursing graduates from the 1965–2016 cohorts and collected their memories. She lovingly restored the first cap worn by our graduates and kept everyone on schedule to produce this book. Her contribution to this history can only be described as extraordinary. She captured the powerful spirit that appeared early in the school's life and that continues to enrich the lives of students, faculty, and graduates today.

To explore the history of the first 50 years, I thought it best to ask the former deans to tell us in their own voices what the school was like during their tenure—how they began, the events that transpired, and their hopes and dreams for the school's future. As a member of the College of Nursing's faculty for more than 30 years, I have worked with hundreds of faculty and students and served with five deans/directors of nursing. I was privileged to know two of the early leaders, UNC Charlotte president Bonnie Cone, MEd, and Professor Elinor Caddell, RN, MSN. Dona knew them, too, and Dean Edith Brocker, RN, MEd, as well.

In working together, the two of us developed a relationship we have come to prize. In collaborating on writing this book we searched for a single voice, a collective "we." We learned to listen to each other and build on each other's insights. Hence, this book is not separated into parts that we wish to attribute to one or the other of us, even though each of us took the primary responsibility for different parts. There may be stylistic differences, but the book as a whole is the product of our joint efforts.

We are grateful for the cooperation, assistance, and support of many persons. Ashley Lopez, a graduate assistant, found the tattered cardboard box and transferred its contents to a safer plastic storage bin and labeled it "Nursing History and Pictures." Upon inquiry, she took us straight to what has become known "The Box."

The staff of the UNC Charlotte J. Murrey Atkins Library gave invaluable assistance. When we met her, we knew that we had found our champion in Somaly Kim Wu, MLIS, Head of Library Technology and Innovation. She helped us navigate the world of publishing and introduced us to John McLeod of the UNC Press Office of Scholarly Publishing. He, in turn, did all the rest necessary to bring our book to life. Ryan Miller of the Atkins Library at UNC Charlotte designed the cover for the book and other library staff, most notably those in the Special Collections and Archives, pulled box after box of archived material for months so that Dona and I, who became known just as "The Nurses," could have everything we needed. A special thanks to Olivia Eanes, Pamela Mason, Alison Wilson, Lolita Rowe, and Tina Wright for supplying us with these archived materials. Thank you to Shannon Homesley and Shannon Dudley of Provost Joan Lorden's office who furnished us with documents that had not yet been archived.

The College/School of Nursing papers cited in the notes are composed of two major groups: The College of Nursing Archives Collection (CON Archives) is found in the Archives of the UNC Charlotte J. Murrey Atkins Library and the

College of Nursing/College of Health and Human Services (CHHS)—School of Nursing historical papers not yet archived (CON/CHHS History) are in the SON director's Suite in the CHHS.

To the students who wrote about their memories and the deans who wrote about the trials and triumphs of their tenures, your contributions provided the foundation for this book about the formative first 50 years. Christian Carballo, RN, MSN, one of our own Niner Nurses gave our manuscript its first read. We also want to express our gratitude to Dr. Dena Evans, interim director of the School of Nursing. Even though she had just come on board, she took a chance on us and provided an editor. A special thank you from Ann to her daughter-in-love, Thea Mayne, for always being there to listen. Dona thanks her patient husband Loy Haney for his support. Thanks to you, our readers, we hope this book will help you fondly remember your years of becoming a "Niner Nurse" at UNC Charlotte.

A Brief History of UNC Charlotte's School of Nursing

Ann Mabe Newman, RN, PhD,
with updates by Dee Baldwin, RN, PhD

On April 17, 1964, the N.C. State Board of Higher Education authorized Charlotte College to offer a four-year program leading to a bachelor of science in nursing degree. Under the direction of UNC Charlotte president Bonnie Cone, Edith Brocker, RN, MEd, was appointed chair of the Department of Nursing, and students enrolled in the spring semester of 1965.

On July 1, 1965, Charlotte College became UNC Charlotte, and the Department of Nursing became the College of Nursing. The start-up costs for the college were estimated to be less than $25,000.[1] Edith Brocker, became the first dean. According to her handwritten reports of the first year, "Things really began to move forward with the hiring of the first faculty member, Miss Elinor Caddell." Our beloved Elinor Caddell, RN, MSN, began the business of nursing education with six students. Over the next quarter of a century, many more students benefited from her teaching. She remains active in the life of the UNC Charlotte School of Nursing (SON).

When Dean Brocker retired in 1972, Dr. Marinell Jernigan, RN, EdD, replaced her as dean and remained in that position until 1977, when Dr. Jernigan returned to full-time teaching and Dr. Louise Schlachter, RN, PhD, then became dean. The college continued to grow and excel and was granted National League for Nursing (NLN) accreditation in December 1974. In 1978, the RN to BSN program was established, and in that same year, the Gamma Iota Chapter of Sigma Theta Tau International was founded. By 1982, the nursing program had expanded to include graduate education, followed by the first specialty track: adult health nursing. In 1984, the Clinical Nurse Specialist (CNS) in Pediatric Nursing was established. Dr. Nancy Langston, RN, PhD, became dean in 1985, and degrees in Psychiatric Mental

Health Nursing, Nursing Administration, and a Nursing and Business Administration dual degree were established. By 1988, the Nurse Anesthesia concentration had been instituted in partnership with the Carolinas Medical Center as an MSN specialty.

From 1993–96, health-related programs and research were identified as top priorities for UNC Charlotte, and the College of Nursing responded by establishing health as a multidisciplinary mission. From 1992 to 2004, Dean Sue Bishop, RN, PhD, led the college through an exciting period of growth. The new College of Health and Human Services (CHHS) building was designed under her guidance, and the College of Nursing was expanded to become the College of Nursing and Health Professions. By 2000, the University Health Commission recommended further expansion in health and human services. Nursing, Kinesiology, Social Work, and Health Behavior and Administration were named departments, and the School of Nursing was named and became the first school organized within a college at UNC Charlotte in 2002. After Dean Bishop's retirement, Dr. Pam Larsen, RN, PhD, the associate dean of the College of Nursing, became the director of the new School of Nursing from 2002–05, followed by Dr. Lucille Travis, RN, PhD, from 2005 to 2007. Dr. Jane Neese, PhD, associate dean of the College of Nursing and Health Professions, served as interim director from 2008–09, when Dr. Dee Baldwin, RN, PhD, assumed the helm as associate dean and director of the School of Nursing. She served from 2009–17, and under her leadership, the school achieved a successful Commission on Collegiate Nursing Education (CCNE) 10-year reaccreditation review of its undergraduate education and master's programs in nursing in 2011. Enhanced national prominence of the school also was achieved as evidenced by a jump in national rankings from 87 to 54 for the Online Graduate programs reported by *US News & World Reports*[2] in 2015 and the school's achievement of a National Center of Excellence[3] designation by the National League for Nursing in the area of Creating Environments that Enhance Student Learning and Professional Development in 2016. The RN-to-BSN program doubled its enrollment in 2015, with an Early Entry option for community college graduates offered in 2016; and the school's new partnership with Carolinas HealthCare Systems led to the Adult Gerontology Acute Care Nurse Practitioner option in the MSN program.

The UNC Charlotte/WCU Dual Doctor of Nursing Practice Degree program was established in 2013 as the school's first doctoral degree. The doctoral program was a joint effort by the schools of nursing at UNC Charlotte and Western Carolina University. Its approval was groundbreaking, as UNC Charlotte became one of the six institutions in the state approved by the University of North Carolina system to offer the DNP degree as a terminal degree. The DNP program received a five-year initial accreditation from the CCNE in September 2016 with Dr. Baldwin serving as the first chief nurse administrator of the dual-degree program.

The School of Nursing Alumni Chapter (SONAC) was named the first academic alumni chapter on UNC Charlotte's campus in 2012 at a notable event to reunite alumni and jump start the organization by sponsoring annual summits. Three years later, at a summit, chapter members approved the concept of recognizing nurses who serve as leaders, experts, scholars, and partners to improve nursing and health care as "Niner Nurses." All alumni now proudly refer to themselves as "Niner Nurses."

A New College of Nursing—Three Special Women Will Bring It to Life

DONA HANEY, RN, MSN

In August 1965, a group of 26 anxious, excited young women gathered for their first session of Ecology of Man 101. This was their very first nursing class, and they were the first nursing cohort in a new nursing program. But long before this class convened, forward-thinking individuals had devised a plan for the College of Nursing to become one of the first four colleges in the University of North Carolina at Charlotte.

The School of Nursing owes a tremendous debt to those who identified the need for baccalaureate-prepared nurses and to those who worked diligently to bring the program into being.

Three women were the program's pioneers: Bonnie Cone, Edith Brocker, and Elinor Caddell. These individuals envisioned the possibility of a four-year nursing program, worked diligently to bring the vision to fruition, and introduced the community to the BSN nurse.

Bonnie Cone, Founder and President of UNC Charlotte

Bonnie Cone lived the history of the University of North Carolina at Charlotte. She grew up in South Carolina and always planned to be a teacher. Cone graduated from Coker College in Hartsville, South Carolina, in 1928, then taught math at high schools in the state. She moved to North Carolina to pursue a master's degree at Duke University, and while there, taught veterans returning from World War II. Upon completion of her master's degree in 1940, Cone took a job in Charlotte at Charlotte Central High School teaching math. The rest is history.

An article in the *Carolina Journal* on July 3, 1973, outlines the first 27 years of the university's history under Cone's leadership:[4]

- In 1946, Cone was at Central High School, Charlotte, North Carolina, teaching a variety of math courses. In addition, she took a part-time position teaching engineering math at the Charlotte Center of the University of North Carolina, a night school housed in Central High to serve World War II veterans going to school on the GI Bill of Rights.
- The following year, she became director of the Charlotte Center.
- In 1949, under Cone's leadership and with the help of many community leaders, the Charlotte Center was converted into Charlotte College, a two-year junior college.
- In 1958, Charlotte College came under the NC Community College system.
- In 1961, the college moved from the old Central High School to a 1,000-acre campus.
- In 1963, Charlotte College became a four-year college.
- In 1965, Charlotte College became a UNC college.

Early in her career, Cone became known as "Miss Bonnie" as she developed personal relationships with students she was teaching. There are numerous stories of the impact she had on the lives of individuals she motivated and guided. Her colleagues described her as a compassionate, caring individual.

The College of Nursing was one of four original colleges planned for the university. Miss Bonnie was instrumental in establishing the UNC Charlotte School of Nursing as evidenced by documents found in the Atkins Library Archives. Miss Bonnie was committed to making this college a reality, or as nurses would say, "birthing the program."

First, the Charlotte College would need approval from the National League for Nursing (NLN) to begin a new college of nursing. This process began long before approval would be sought for the new program. The first step would be for the NLN to conduct an on-site visit, which was done from June 12–14, 1963. The NLN representatives met with Cone, Dean Bill McCoy of the Education Department, and selected faculty members representing disciplines pertinent to undergraduate education, in addition to about 35 representatives of local hospitals, schools of nursing, the Mecklenburg County Health Department, the UNC Chapel Hill School of Nursing, the NC Board of Health, the NC Board of Nurse Registration and Nurse Education, the Duke Endowment, and the NC State Board of Higher Education. Findings of this visit included the following:

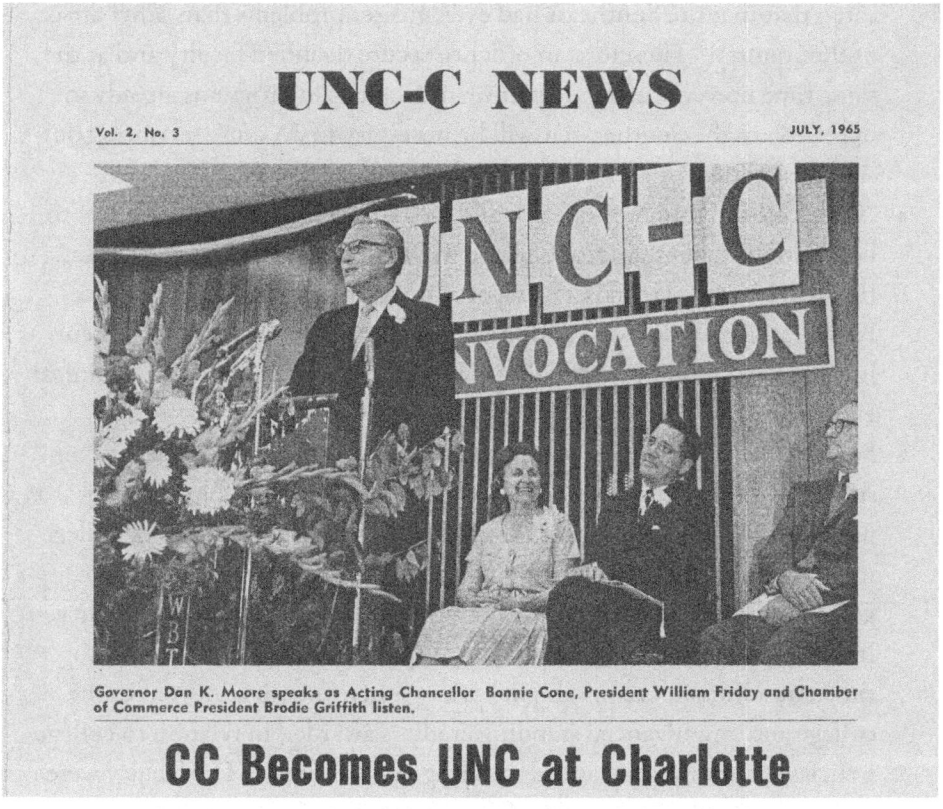

UNC-C NEWS

Vol. 2, No. 3   JULY, 1965

Governor Dan K. Moore speaks as Acting Chancellor Bonnie Cone, President William Friday and Chamber of Commerce President Brodie Griffith listen.

CC Becomes UNC at Charlotte

Charlotte College becomes UNC Charlotte.

- "There was evidence that the development of a baccalaureate program in nursing had been given a great deal of thought by President Cone and other college personnel. It was also evident that the representatives present at the group meeting had been brought into the pre-planning activities. The interest and enthusiasm of this group of community representatives was impressive as was their understanding of baccalaureate education in nursing and their desire for a quality program at this level."
- College resources were noted in most instances to be more than adequate. However, it was noted that the Biology Department did not have any courses in anatomy and physiology, which would be "essential for a nursing program."
- Another obstacle was recruitment of faculty. "Since nursing personnel prepared for teaching in collegiate programs are in extremely short supply, it can be anticipated that recruitment of qualified faculty for this program will be a major problem." Statistics regarding shortages indi-

cated that that the Southeast had even greater problems than other areas of the country. "Therefore, in order to secure qualified faculty and at the same time prevent further depletion of faculties in programs already in operation in the Southeast, it will be necessary to do some recruiting outside the region."

- "Charlotte has numerous health and welfare agencies and there seems to be no doubt that Charlotte College will have access to clinical facilities that will be adequate in both extent and variety for student experiences." However, the school was cautioned that with two other schools present in the area, it might be difficult to meet all the students' needs for clinical experiences.

- Some of the comments made by community representatives led the consultant to note that "there will undoubtedly be pressure for the college to offer baccalaureate education for graduates of hospital and junior college nursing programs." It was suggested that they wait until the basic program was well developed before taking on this additional responsibility. It was also noted that "Graduate nurse applicants should be subject to the same admission requirements as any other student admitted to the college and any advanced standing credit is awarded in relation to college policies for granting advanced standing in other areas." The faculty were encouraged to devise a means of assuring that graduate nursing students acquired a baccalaureate level of competence in nursing by such means as challenge examinations, special projects, or completion of the courses offered to basic nursing students.[5] The following year, in May 1964, Cone signed the application to establish a school of nursing.[6]

As plans for nursing proceeded, Miss Bonnie was instrumental in selecting the program's leader. She recruited Edith Brocker, RN, MEd, assistant director of the School of Nursing at Duke University to be dean of the new program.

In the planning process, Miss Bonnie met with the NC Board of Nurse Registration and Nursing Education on January 27, 1965, to present a proposal for the School of Nursing. Edith Brocker was invited to join the team for the presentation. In a follow-up communication of this meeting, Priscilla D. Balance, chair of the NC Board of Nurse Registration and Nursing Education, reported that the board met on January 28, 1965, and granted provisional accreditation to the Department of Nursing, Charlotte College, effective September 1, 1965.

In July 1965, Charlotte College became part of the University of North Carolina system and became the University of North Carolina at Charlotte. That same year, Miss Bonnie was recognized as a Distinguished Citizen of Charlotte by the Charlotte Civitans. She was acknowledged to be the catalyst behind the struggle to establish Charlotte College, to build it up, and to make it a part of the UNC system. She also received the Distinguished Citizen of North Carolina award in 1965.

Her former pastor, Rev. George Heaton of Myers Park Baptist Church, Charlotte, said of her: "This woman, Bonnie Cone, was possessed of a dream and she possessed those qualities where she gave of herself to something so big that it will require decades for people to finish that which she initiated among us."[7]

In 1965, Miss Bonnie became the vice chancellor for Student Affairs and Community relations, a position she held until her retirement in June 1973. At her retirement, the Student Union was renamed the Bonnie Cone Student Union. Even then, she continued to work part time with the Development Office and the UNC Charlotte Foundation.

In 1979, UNC Charlotte awarded Cone an honorary Doctor of Humanities—the university's highest award. During the awards ceremony, she was acknowledged as a visionary and a hard worker who brought the university and the College of Nursing into being. The College of Nursing continues to be a recipient of the vision and diligence of Dr. Cone.

Although she never married and had no children, as she neared retirement, Bonnie described the school as her family. Members of the university felt the same way. Administration, faculty, and alumni developed a plan to bury her on campus near the Van Landingham Glen. Dr. James H. Woodward, chancellor emeritus, shared the plan with her. Cone died in 2003 at the age of 95 and is buried on the campus of UNC Charlotte. The inscription on her tombstone reads, "Bonnie E. Cone, June 22, 1907–March 24, 2009, Founder of the University of North Carolina at Charlotte." It includes a quote from Edward Everett Hale (1822–1909), an American author, historian, and Unitarian minister:

> I am only one, But I am one,
> I cannot do everything, but I can do something.
> What I can do, I ought to do and what I might do,
> By the Grace of God, I will.

An engraving of a stylized pine cone, an early symbol of UNC Charlotte, is at the bottom of the inscription.

Edith Brocker, First Department Chair of School of Nursing (1964–1972)

Edith Brocker was well prepared to lead the new school of nursing. She graduated from the University of Pennsylvania with a diploma in nursing in 1930. She worked for several years in the hospital setting and then developed an interest in public health nursing. Brocker returned to school and earned a Certificate in Public Health Nursing from the College of William and Mary in Richmond, Virginia, in 1943 and a BS in Public Health Nursing in 1944. She held a variety of public health positions before returning to her home state of North Carolina in 1946 to become the supervising public health nurse for the District Health Department in Chapel Hill. In this position, she also took on the role of an ad hoc instructor in Public Health Nursing for the University of North Carolina at Chapel Hill. Her interest in nursing education led her to obtain her master's in nursing education in 1951.

In 1954, Brocker became president of the North Carolina State Nurses Association. An article in the *Tar Heel Nurse* in December 1954 contained a number of tributes from colleagues:

> She is a thorough thinker. She thinks through situations before making a conclusion. . . . She listens well. When she speaks, she has something to say. . . . People wait for what she has to say.

> She has a wonderful sense of humor, and she tells her little stories with a twinkle in her eye.

> Definitely a leader. . . . Sincere. . . . She has high principles and she lives her beliefs. She has dignity and poise.[8]

Brocker was also known for her hospitality. As one colleague noted, she "entertains often, takes pride in her cooking[,] . . . and is a bold and able gardener of both flowers and vegetables. She enjoys the good things of life. The wild birds around her home are her pets."

In 1953, Rosario A. Ortis, a visiting nurse from Manila, Philippines, described her experience with Brocker this way: "I shall never forget the very warm welcome I received from Mrs. Brocker, the Supervising Nurse of the District Health Department," she said of their meeting at the Raleigh railroad station the Sunday evening she arrived in Charlotte.

> My feeling of uncertainty in the new environment was greatly relieved when Mrs. Brocker approached me as I got off the train, my hands full with suitcase

and coats. Immediately Mrs. Brocker and her friend took my luggage from me, shook my hand, and introduced themselves. "You are staying with us, if you so desire," Mrs. Brocker said. I was immediately relieved. I was so deeply touched by her friendliness that I accepted without hesitation the invitation. . . . That very pleasant welcome I shall never forget, for it made me feel at home right away in North Carolina, and gave me an impression that my stay would be a very enjoyable one, which it certainly was.[9]

In 1955, Brocker became an instructor in Public Health Nursing at Duke University School of Nursing. In 1957, she became the assistant dean of the Duke University School of Nursing.

While at Duke, she assisted Dr. Cone as she prepared the application to the North Carolina Board of Nurse Registration and Nursing Education for the new School of Nursing at the University of North Carolina at Charlotte. Dr. Cone asked Edith Brocker to be the first director of the UNC Charlotte School of Nursing. In 1964, Brocker began commuting from Duke to perform preliminary work for the new program. In early 1965, she moved to Charlotte and assumed her new position full time.

Her gifts of hospitality were called upon frequently in her new position as head of the nursing program in Charlotte. She hosted many social events for the students at her home, some on multiple days to make sure that classes did not interfere and that all students got the opportunity to participate.

Gerri Brady, RN, MSN, a faculty member from 1968–77, said Brocker "cared a great deal about faculty, listened carefully. She was very supportive. She called me into her office one day and said, 'Here, I made you a crying towel.'" Brady says this was an appropriate gesture as she was constantly "crying on her shoulder that we could do better than we are doing."[10]

Joyce Lowder, RN, MSN, faculty member from 1967–70, also expressed her admiration. "I have very fond memories of Dr. Edith Brocker, from my first interview with her. Her gentle spirit, coupled with high expectations for the growth of the program, was most impressive and appreciated! She had dreams of the success of this program. She worked incessantly, not easy when the nursing program was small compared to other departments. I respected her so much that I decided to stitch a pair of lace gloves for her. I finished them, late at night, before the Christmas party the next day. I placed them out to look at them . . . and found that I had made two right-hand gloves!!!! Yes, I did take out the stitches and fixed the problem, on time!"[11]

With the new program at Charlotte College, later UNC Charlotte SON, in the early planning stages, Brocker penned some "Basic Factors for Consideration."[12] The following are excerpts from this document:

- We have attempted to set up a four-year academic year plan. There is no other in North Carolina at this moment.
- My belief about nursing—stated far too simply—is that a nurse's fortune is in her hands, but her hands must be directed by a disciplined mind and a compassionate heart, and her portfolio of knowledge must be a growing and changing part of her life.
- We hope to offer both men and women a basic, generic program with a major in nursing. A major in nursing will offer skills in patient care—sick children, sick adults—in home, hospital, and health agencies (medical, surgical, psychiatric). In order to understand the abnormal, they need know something of the well person—from preconception to premortuary. We will emphasize "service and "care" in their highest meaning.
- With chronic illness and increased hospitalizations, we can expect a different level of home care program—something we have not dreamed of yet.
- I very much want more ladies in our legislature to help us with our laws, and we need nurse lawyers.
- We have to prepare a person who can be useful right here in Charlotte, east, west, and middle North Carolina (able to nurse our white folk, our negroes, Indians, and foreigners from other states and countries). . . . I don't believe we can be a *university* and prepare people to be provincial.
- I believe that there must be one course in nursing in the first year to strengthen or make use of the student's motivation to be a nurse and to make contact with the nursing faculty. I don't want too much nursing in the first year so that if a person wishes to change the major, he or she can now move easily into another program. One year of maturity before going into nursing is good.
- Now these are my purposes, some of my problems, some of the excitement, a bit of my philosophy. Now how do we get all of this into a program that can be taught to young people's hands, hearts, and minds at Charlotte College?

no uniform - no cap - no pin - all symbols have
to created.

1) We have attempted to set up a 4-yr academic year
plan - there is no other in N.C. at this moment
This means that it is less expensive - We have an open quota-

2) I have my heart set on a different way of
teaching nursing - (we can save that for
another Cur. Comm. mtg.) But I am hoping very
much that as we teach the nursing skills of
patient care - we can also share some of your knowledge
and basic understanding of the meaning of community,
in its broadest sense.

My own belief about nsg - stated far too simply - is
that a nurse's fortune in her hands - but her hands
must be directed by a disciplined mind and a
compassionate heart - & that her portfolio of knowledge
must be a growing and changing part of her life.

We hope to offer both men & women a basic - generic
program & a major in nursing -
A major that will offer skills in patient care -
sick children, sick adults - in home, hospitals and
health agencies - (medical, surg. psychiatric patient
& in order to understand the abnormal, they need to something
of the well person - from the preconception to the
post-mortuary, we will emphasize "service" & "care")
in their highest meaning - Our clinical instructors
will be skilled practitioners because we believe in the laying
on of hands.

Documents containing notes for consideration from Edith Brocker.

Elinor Caddell, RN, MSN, Second Faculty Member (1965–1989)

In 1965, when Elinor Caddell was teaching nursing at Duke University and had the opportunity to come to UNC Charlotte, she was coming home. Elinor spent most of her youth in Charlotte and graduated from Central High School. Her vision after high school was to go to medical school, but it was not financially feasible.

She heard that Charlotte Memorial Hospital was starting a new nursing school and that free tuition and a stipend were available for those who signed up for the cadet corp. Due to World War II, the government was offering to provide nursing education in exchange for two years' service in any of the armed services after graduation. She enrolled in the Charlotte Memorial School of Nursing as a cadet nurse in 1941 at the age of 17. She was an outstanding student. Then, in her senior year, the school needed additional instructors for fundamental students. Elinor describes that they "put me in a white uniform and had me checking off skills for freshman students."

When the war ended in 1945, she was relieved of the responsibly to go into the service. So instead, she stayed on at the hospital for another year and worked in general medicine. During this time, she took courses at Queens University in Charlotte in preparation to enter the baccalaureate nursing program at Duke University.

Because there was a need for nurses to teach nursing, Duke University offered a grant for a two-year program to provide a BS in nursing education. Elinor was in the first class of that program. She came back to Charlotte Memorial Hospital School of Nursing to teach. In her first year, she taught anatomy and physiology, chemistry, sociology, microbiology, and pharmacology.

She taught at Charlotte Memorial Hospital School of Nursing for 10 years and then returned to Duke University to obtain a master's degree in nursing. Upon graduation, she was asked to teach at Duke University, and she did so from 1960–65.

When Dr. Cone asked Edith Brocker to take the position of director at UNC Charlotte College of Nursing, Brocker said, "I will come if I can bring Elinor with me." Elinor left Duke University in 1965 to take her place as the second UNC Charlotte SON faculty member. For her first two years, she taught all medical-surgical courses, including medical-surgical nursing, leadership, and critical care. In addition to teaching, she was also very active in organizational activities and attended many committee meetings. A professor noted that she attended many meetings, and she responded, "There are only two of us, so each of us attends one-half of all committees."[13]

"Change is exciting, if you like what you are doing," Elinor said of her work, and it was "so exciting developing and creating the school."

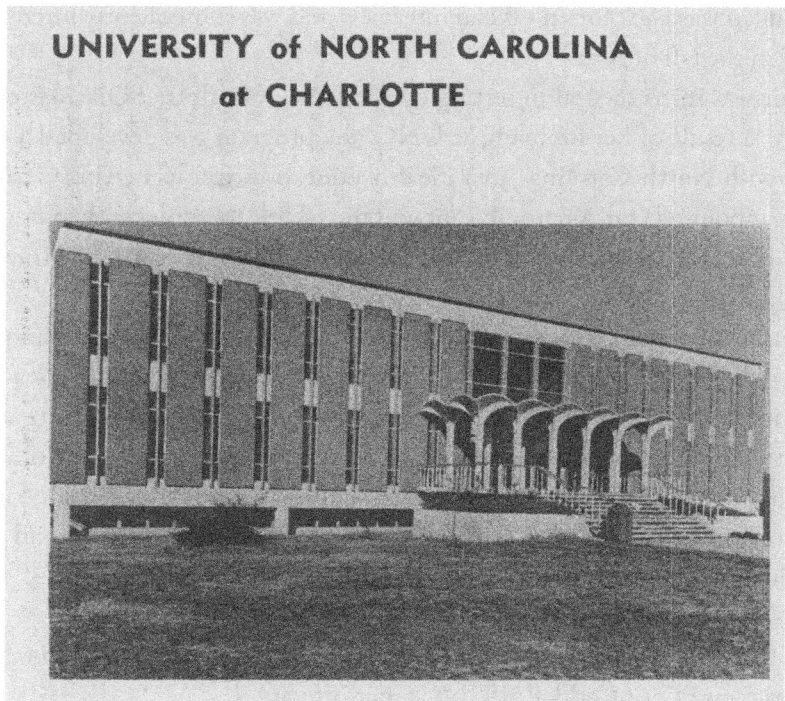

Kennedy Building.

At the time, there were only four classroom buildings: Bernard, Garinger, Denny, and Kennedy. The campus also included the J. Murrey Atkins Library and the Student Union. "The buildings we taught in were one story. There were no paved parking lots, parking was plentiful, often easy to park very close to our building."

Part of Elinor's job was to counsel RNs about getting their BSN degrees. She was also instrumental in the ongoing recruitment of faculty to meet the needs of a growing student body. Elinor identified UNC Charlotte SON graduates who would be good candidates for such positions. "I was always looking out for those individuals who would do a good job," she said. Many early graduates-turned-faculty remember getting a call from Elinor with a job offer.

Sue Head (class of '71) was a faculty member from 1971–74 and 1976–93. She recalled, "Elinor was intuitive, identified those who had gifts and talents, and she instilled in them the confidence that they could do it."

Ruth Mauldin, RN, MSN, a faculty member from 1970–96, told a story about how a visiting friend left the school with a job offer. "In the spring of 1972, my friend and former classmate at the University of Alabama Nursing School master's program, Dr. Marinell Jernigan, came to visit; and while she was there, Caddell came by to talk with her about the job of dean of the College of Nursing. Soon,

Dr. Jernigan was back for an official interview and was subsequently hired as dean starting in the fall of 1972."[14]

Elinor was instrumental in setting up the UNC Charlotte SON master's program. As a result of her lobbying at UNC, the program was developed as a joint project with North Carolina Area Health Education Centers (AHEC) and Elinor was appointed coordinator. Elinor and the Charlotte students then traveled to Chapel Hill twice a week for coursework. For the first two years, they traveled by small plane, then later by van.

The time came for UNC Charlotte to have its own MSN program. Elinor wrote the plan for the new program and was instrumental in selecting its first leader.

The impact of Elinor Caddell on the history of the College of Nursing at UNC Charlotte cannot be adequately described. She has educated thousands of individuals and influenced the development of the college. Although she retired in 1989, Elinor continues to be a part of the school and the lives of students and alumni through her generous contributions to support life-long learning and nursing scholarship.

The following are some of the memories that have been recorded to reflect on the impact on Elinor Caddell at UNC Charlotte SON.

Joyce Lowder, who was the fourth member of the faculty and taught from 1967–70, describes her interactions with Elinor this way:

> We must have looked like Mutt and Jeff, as she was tall and I was, well, petite. She was tall in more ways than stature! She shared her knowledge, compassion, encouragement, and expertise with me at a time when I really needed it. Her wisdom, common sense, and professionalism was a blessing! There were times when we needed lunch, and she would invite me to join her and her dear mother on the front porch for a bologna and pickle sandwich. . . . She will always hold a special place in my heart! She has had an unforgettable impact on nursing, UNC-C CON, students, patients, and me![15]

Janet Kale Hunt (class of '69), reflected,

> UNC Charlotte's nursing program was almost brand new in the fall of 1965. I was in the second class of students who would graduate in 1969. Elinor Caddell brought together a few students to design the first uniforms and caps. She was not only an excellent teacher and role model, but also a good artist who brought our ideas to life by sketching the designs we suggested. The result, in keeping with university colors, was a forest-green dress with a detachable white apron and a simple white cap.[16]

Dona Harton Haney (class of '69) said, "Elinor taught me every semester of my clinical courses. I continue to count Elinor Caddell as my mentor and very special friend."[17]

In addition to personal praise, Elinor received much public recognition during her career, receiving the following awards:

- UNC Charlotte Teaching Excellence Award (1970)
- Outstanding Nursing Educator, presented by the NC Nurses Association (1990)
- Distinguished Alumni Award, Carolinas College of Health Sciences (2006)
- Honorary Alumni Award, UNC Charlotte School of Nursing Alumni (2015)

Elinor has a sincere dedication to ongoing education and the importance of research. With this in mind, she created the Elinor Caddell Faculty Research Award in 1990. The award provides funds for faculty to assist with costs to further their research. To date, 12 faculty members have received this award. Each recipient is grateful for the recognition of their research efforts and the assistance to complete their project.

In a recent interview, Elinor commented on the paths taken and those not taken, as well as the journey. When asked if she regretted not becoming a physician, she said no, but that she does wish she had gotten a doctorate in education, "I am all about education, I wish I had taken the time to get it done." She has seen many changes in nursing care over her career and believes not all of them were for the better. Technology, for instance, "has taken away from the closeness of the nurse-patient relationship." As for what she takes the most pride in, Elinor says it was teaching. "I loved it when students 'caught on.'"[18]

Dr. Cone, Edith Brocker, and Elinor Caddell are three strong individuals who invested their lives in UNC Charlotte SON. The school's growth and success over its first 50 years are a testament to their talents and drive.

The First Students (Classes of 1968 and 1969)

This first group of students consisted of 20 freshmen and six sophomores. They were all from North Carolina and all were female. Two were African American. They were all going for a college degree at a time when a majority of individuals obtained no more than a high school diploma.

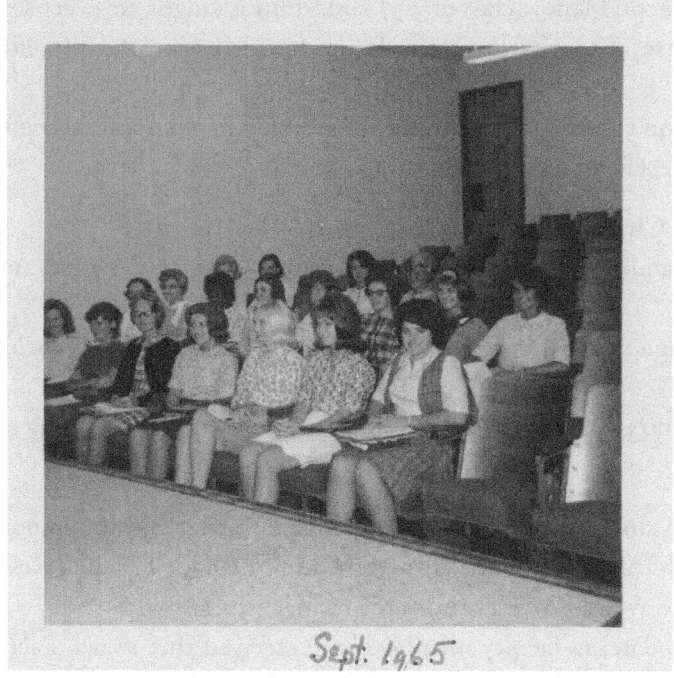

Sept. 1965

Nursing students, 1965.

When I graduated from high school in 1965, 12% of men and only 7.4% of women in the United States had completed four or more years of college. At that time, having a college degree was a ticket to upward mobility. My parents were working-class people, and I was the first person in my father's family to attend college.[19]

This first year, there were no traditions, no uniforms, and only two faculty members—Edith Brocker, dean, and Elinor Caddell, professor. Under normal circumstances, there would only be a freshman class, but since nursing had not been offered before, sophomores at the university were allowed to join the program.

After several weeks of class, the sophomores, who were taking their first medical-surgical nursing class, were ready to begin clinicals, but the newly designed uniform was not yet delivered. The students wore an interim uniform made available by Eugene Smith, RN, MSN, director of Nursing at Charlotte Memorial Hospital (and the husband of Vera Smith, RN, MSN, who would become the third UNC Charlotte SON faculty member). He had located a supply of white, "standard uniforms" (perhaps like those worn by cafeteria staff), which the students wore until the new uniforms were available.

Every nurse remembers her first day of clinicals, but for this group of students, it was particularly exciting. Gloria Johnson (class of '68) shared that, "On my very first day of clinical, I saw a man grab the handrail, and sink to the floor. I quickly ran to get my instructor, Elinor Caddell, and she started CPR and saved the life of a physician. She was a hero to me and made me realize the impact a nurse can have on lives."[20]

The freshmen were excited to hear what the sophomores were doing in clinicals, often asking, "What did you do?" To which one upperclassman responded, "We took TPRs." Lowerclassmen had to ask, "What's that?" because they did not yet understand the clinical nursing lingo.

The new uniforms arrived and were dedicated at a special service, which included a presentation by Elinor Caddell on "The Significance of the Uniform" and a presentation by Bonnie Cone, acting chancellor on "The Place of the Department of Nursing in the University Complex." The most memorable part of the dedication was a prayer by Dr. Loy Witherspoon. As one student remembers, "He blessed every piece of the uniform twice—the dress, the apron, the cap, the shoes, the white hose—everything except our underwear."[21] Despite diligent efforts to find the prayer for this book, we sadly report it was not in the archives.

Nursing students were among the first UNC Charlotte students to live in a dormitory. At the same time the UNC Charlotte SON program was starting, Charlotte Memorial Hospital was phasing out its three-year program and the Central Piedmont Community College was beginning its associate's degree in nursing program. This resulted in dorm space being available on the CMC campus. Janet Kale Hunt (class of '69) recalled that, "The dorm housed female nursing students from UNC Charlotte as well as students with other healthcare specialties (radiology technology, medical technology, etc.). We cooked meals in electric popcorn poppers, hung drinks out the window in pillow cases to get them cool, and pierced each other's ears."[22] While non-nursing students were envious of those individuals who lived in the dorms, the dorms were 30 minutes from campus. All students commuted to campus.

Even though UNC Charlotte was a commuter school, sports and student activities were a part of campus life. Nursing students were involved in all of it. Joyce Edwards and Susan Allen were cheerleaders. Susan was also involved in the student court and became the first female student judge.

Other students describe similar moments during their early clinical experiences:[23]

- A little boy, who was badly burned, died from a related infection.
- A man was so badly burned that he looked like a skeleton.

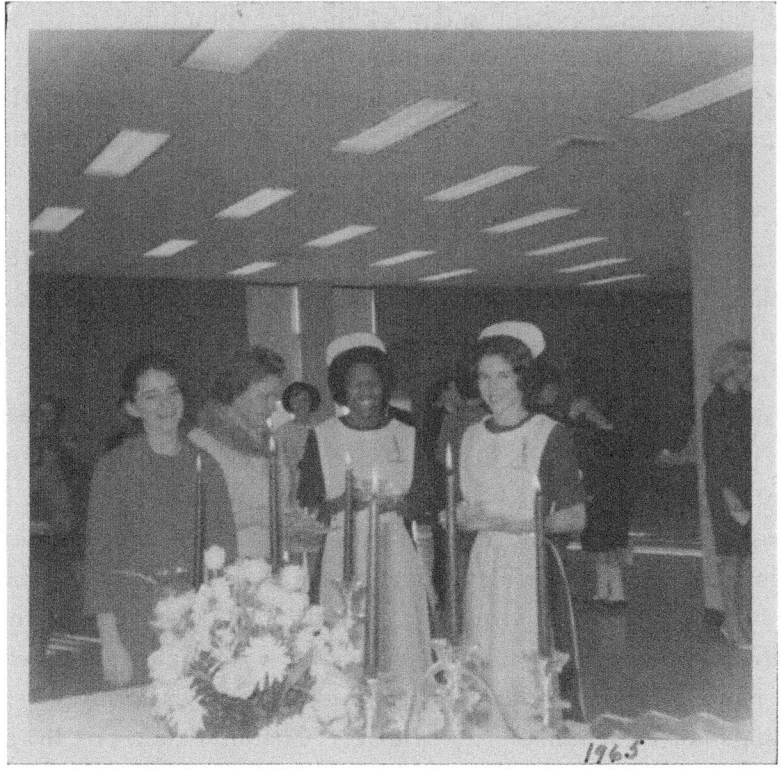

Beth Donnelly and Naomi Fleming proudly wear their uniforms
at the Dedication of the Uniforms ceremony, 1966.

- A woman died in the ER from a hemorrhage (esophageal varices).
- A man came in with terrible injuries; he was in his car when it was struck by a train.
- A young man in his 20s experienced a traumatic brain injury when the truck tire he was filling with air exploded. He survived, but had lasting issues, so his mother took care of him. He later attended his nurse's wedding.

During the turbulent 1960s, it was easy for young Americans to feel unsettled and conflicted. The country was divided on key issues of the time: the war in Vietnam, women's equality, and racial discrimination. Janet Kale (class of '69) recalls the time that she was assigned to care for an African American man in the cardiac unit. "He was clearly distressed to see a young white woman coming to bathe him, and he said something to me about my not wanting to do this because he was black.

I distinctly remember saying, 'I'm not like that.' He became more at ease, and we proceeded with a comfortable degree of mutual understanding."[24]

Barbara Baker Mirgon (class of '69) said, "Being exposed to happenings that I had never experienced in my sheltered life actually helped me grow and not only respect myself, but other people, no matter what the circumstances were."[25]

Other experiences were lessons learned, according to Shelia Frieze Nance (class of '69). "One thing that stayed with me all these years is my OR experience. I was in surgery with Dr. Robicsek and scared to death. He took the time to have me look closely at the patient's lungs. They were black due to smoking. I never smoked. I have told others what I saw throughout my years of practice."[26]

"I remember my first patient, a lady with a leg fracture," recalled Dona Haney (class of '69). "My clinical began at 4 o'clock in the afternoon, and this patient agreed to have her bath at that time. Due to my inexperience, it took me three hours to do this bath. Later in my career as a clinical instructor I would tell this story to ease students' anxieties. I think that helped those students understand that everything does not go as planned."[27]

One nursing student discovered a problem with her hearing while practicing with her stethoscope. She could not hear heart and breath sounds. This was long before the introduction of the American Disabilities Act, which might have found an accommodation for her, but she simply changed her major from nursing to psychology.

Nursing students at the UNC Charlotte College of Nursing were trained to be leaders. At the time, most students thought that meant becoming a head nurse someday. Looking back 50 years, we understand, once again, that our instructors had a vision for us. The first group of students did become leaders in clinical practice, education, and administration. They were head nurses, shift supervisors, quality managers, book authors, and educators. This group were leaders in medical surgical, mental health, long-term care, and physician offices settings. All are now retired from professional nursing practice.

CHAPTER ONE

The Beginning Years

Edith Brocker, RN, MEd,
Founding Dean of the College of Nursing, 1965–1972

Dona H. Haney, RN, MSN

In January 1965, the North Carolina Board of Nursing approved the creation of a nursing program at UNC Charlotte. That same month, Edith Perryman Brocker accepted the invitation of Dr. Bonnie Cone, the founder of UNC Charlotte, to lead the program. She immediately began the work of implementing the program and hired a faculty member, Elinor Caddell, RN, MSN, who would start in the fall. Her task was to select students from among the applicants to the nursing program, secure clinical laboratory sites for students to practice the delivery of nursing care to patients, and design nursing courses for the term beginning in September.

An announcement[1] in the local newspaper and a write-up[2] in the North Carolina Board of Nursing's list of approved schools served as the program's first solicitations for students. In her first annual report,[3] Dean Brocker noted that referrals also came from a variety of sources:

- One was referred by Herman Hechenbleikner, PhD ("Dr. Heck"), who was her academic advisor and a biology professor. The student knew that she liked sciences but did not see herself in education or in medicine. Her advisor recommended that she check into the nursing program that was just getting started.
- One was encouraged by her guidance counselor. "With your grades, if you want to be a nurse you should go to a four-year program."[4]
- Several had families or friends who understood that the "future of nursing was moving toward requiring a four-year degree."
- Two describe family situations that made a commuter program preferable

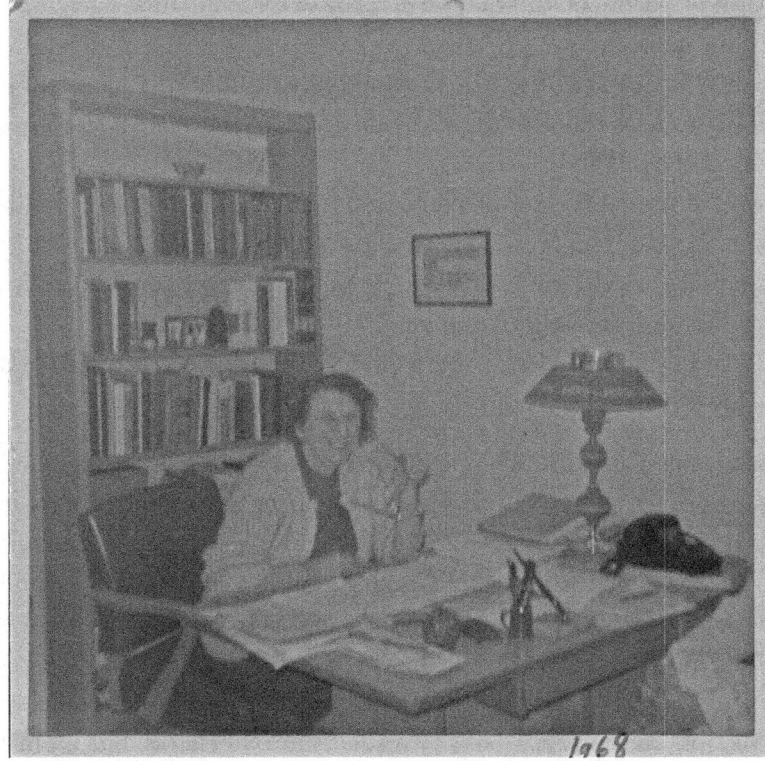

Edith Brocker, first dean of the School of Nursing.

to the residential program required by the diploma programs. Although there were many commuter students in the nursing program, housing was available.

Finding qualified students was not a problem. Dean Brocker spent time researching a variety of potential clinical laboratory sites where students could practice delivering nursing care. The community was very receptive to being a part of the new nursing program. Charlotte Memorial Hospital and the Mecklenburg County Health Department quickly signed on to offer clinical experiences for these students.

An article from the *Charlotte Observer* on February 3, 1965, proclaimed "Nurse Training Program Activated"[5] and offered these details:

- Edith P. Brocker, former assistant dean of the Duke University School of Nursing, began work as the first chairman of the college's department of nursing.
- Officials at Charlotte Memorial Hospital and the Mecklenburg County

Health Department said they were ready to sign affiliation agreements
with the new school.

- The NC Board of Nurse Registry and Nursing Education granted "provisional accreditation" to the school, a necessary assessment to ensure
  safety to the public.
- Eugene J. Smith, director of Nursing at Charlotte Memorial Hospital
  said at an afternoon press conference: "Whatever facilities we have at
  Memorial Hospital are available to nursing students from UNC Charlotte. We want the college students."
- Dr. Maurice Kamp, Mecklenburg County Health director, pledged the
  Health Department's support.

Another article found in "The Box" in the School of Nursing described the infant nursing program at UNC Charlotte: "Building a nursing program from the
ground up can be quite a chore, but UNC Charlotte has a qualified architect in
Edith Brocker." The article describes the education and experience of Dean Brocker
and how the program is "unique in Charlotte in that it is a four-year academic program leading to a B.S. degree with a major in nursing" and that the graduates will be
eligible to become RNs or to take master's degree work in specialized fields. It cites
that the school "currently has only 23 students in two classes, but Dean Brocker
envisions the day when they will have 40 in the freshman class."[6]

The infancy of the nursing program is documented in three years of annual reports, which are located in the Atkins Library archives. A review of the "First Annual Report of the Department of Nursing at UNC-C" (September 1965–June
1966)[7] lists some of the major activities. Dean Brocker offered an outline of these
activities in her report:

Related to curriculum:

- A complete curriculum pattern (for four years) was designed and pre-
  sented to the Curriculum Committee and faculty, and was approved.
- Contracts for clinical facilities were written, signed and incorporated in
  the accreditation reports to the NC Board of Nursing.
- Three major reports were prepared and submitted to the NC Board of
  Nursing. Provisional accreditation was granted for 1965–66.
- Material was prepared for the UNC Charlotte course catalog.

Regarding advisement of students:

- Faculty participated in advisement and registration day for each term.
- Faculty have had both scheduled and open-office hours for academic advisement for all students in nursing throughout the year.

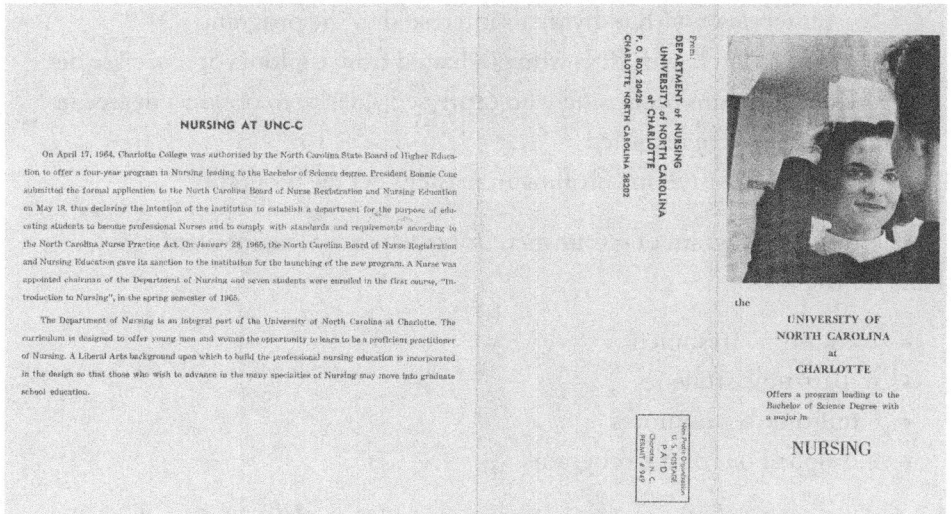

First brochure of the College of Nursing, exterior.

Faculty-student projects:

- Student-nurse uniforms were designed and selected.
- A dedication service for the school uniform was held.
- The student-nurse club was organized.

Recruitment of students and teachers:

- A brochure about the Department of Nursing was produced.
- Faculty speaking at schools was initiated to recruit students
- Letters, telephone calls, and office conferences consisted of:

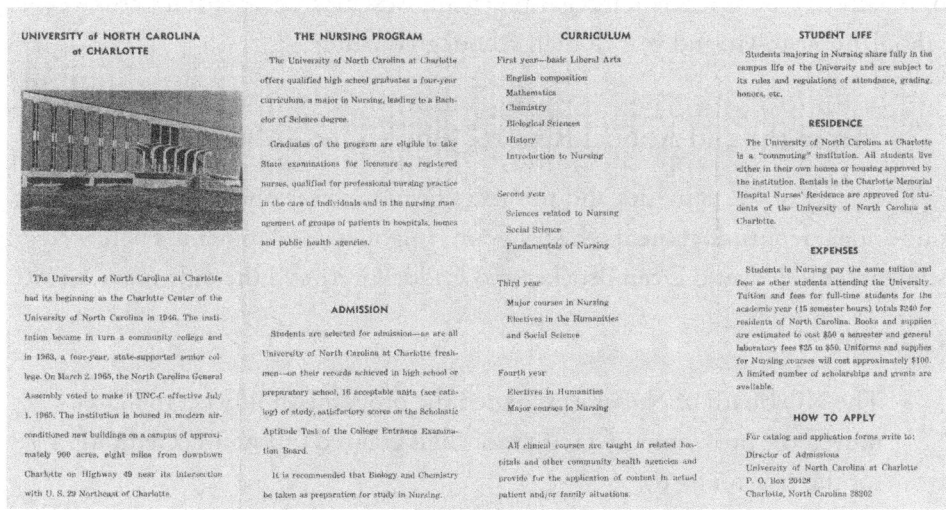

First brochure of the College of Nursing, interior.

* 75 interviews with individuals interested in the program
* 23 interviews, with RNs who graduated from diploma or associate degree programs in nursing who expressed a desire to obtain a degree in nursing, were recorded
* 4 nurses assisted in enrolling in master's degree programs

- Constant program of recruitment for teachers was maintained.

Data for the year:

- 20 full-time freshmen
- 10 part-time students
- 6 full-time sophomores
- 4 dropped out of the program

Newspaper clippings from this year suggest that Dean Brocker was, herself, a resource for the university. She spoke at many nursing and community organizations and was identified by these groups and in the news media as "the director of the new UNC Charlotte School of Nursing."[8]

A copy of *A Survey of Nursing Education Needs*,[9] a report to the NC Board of Higher Education, was also found in the Atkins Library archives. The questions in the survey included: "How many students graduated from your program in 1965? (Total? No. of male? No. of Negroes?)" Of course, the answer to all three questions was none as the program had just begun and graduated no students. However, Dean Brocker reported a maximum of 40 new students expected in the fall of 1966, and that the maximum number of students she would like to admit each year would be 60–70. Attached to the report was a handwritten list of all students enrolled as of March 31, 1966, with details regarding name, sex, race, age, marital status, year in school, home town, and year of high school graduation.

From the 2nd Annual Report (June 1, 1966–May 31, 1967)[10]

While many of the activities and priorities begun in year one continued, the second annual report documents the program's ongoing development. There were 52 students enrolled, and Dean Brocker and Caddell were still the only nurse faculty.

Curriculum:

- The NC Board of Nursing evaluated the program on July 14, 1966, removed the provisional accreditation, and granted full state accreditation for the year 1966–67.

LIST OF STUDENTS

(1)　　Name	(2)　Sex	(3)　Race	(4)　Age	(5)　Marital Status	(6)　Year in School	(7)　Home Base	(8)　Year of HS Graduation
Baker, Barbara	f	w	1947	S	Fr.	Charlotte, N.C.	1965
Baucom, Carol	f	w	1947	S	Fr.	Polkton, N.C.	1965
Beverly, Patricia	f	w	1947	S	fr.	Charlotte, N.C.	1965
Champion, June	f	w.	1947	S	fr.	Charlotte, N.C.	1965
Edwards, Joyce	f	w	1947	S	fr.	Charlotte, N.C	1965
Jesperman, Vickie	f	w.	1947	S.	fr.	Winston-Salem, NC	1965
Freeze, Sheila	f	w	1946	S	fr.	China Grove, NC	1965
Norton, Donna	f	w	1946	S	fr.	Charlotte, N.C.	1965
Ingram, Barbara	f	w	1947	S	fr.	Kannapolis, N.C.	1965
Kale, Janet	f	w	1947	S	fr.	Charlotte, N.C.	1965
Ledford, Kathleen	f	w	1946	S	fr.	Waxhaw, N.C.	65
Madison, Wanda	f	w	1947	S	fr.	Olin, N.C.	1965
McBiff, Patricia	f	c.	1945	S	fr.	Charlotte, N.C.	1962
Roberts, Gloria	f	w	1947	S	fr.	Monroe, N.C.	1965
Roberts, Melody	f	w	1947	S	fr.	Tabor City, N.C.	1965
Smith, Linda	f	w	1947	S.	fr.	Charlotte, N.C.	1965
Alexander, Dorothy	f	w	1946	S	Soph.	Landis, N.C.	1964
Donnelly, Sarah	f	w	1945	S	Soph.	Concord, N.C.	1963
Fleming, Norma	f	c	1945	S	Soph	Morganton, N.C.	1963
Pearce, Marilyn	f	w	1946	S	Soph.	Charlotte, N.C.	1964
Powell, Patricia	f	w	1946	S	Soph	Charlotte, N.C.	1964
Wilkinson, Gloria	f	w	1946	S	Soph.	Charlotte, N.C.	1964

(Attach additional sheet as necessary)

Listing of first students for state report.

- Contracts with Charlotte Memorial Hospital and the Mecklenburg County Health Department were signed.

Faculty-Student Extracurriculars:

- "Social Standards" were developed, relating particularly to the appropriate wearing of the uniform.
- There was increased involvement of faculty in student-nurse club activities.
- The faculty entertained the juniors at a formal candlelight dinner with Dr. Bonnie Cone as the honored guest.
- On November 14 and 16, Hogan's Stew dinners were held for all students.
- Recruitment of students and faculty.
- A new brochure was published.
- Faculty spoke about the program at many professional and civic organizations.
- Letters of inquiry were received from 77 individuals:

  * 58 asking about the four-year program
  * 19 RNs seeking information about the BSN program

- At least five phone calls a week came from RNs who had graduated from diploma or associated degree programs seeking BSN degrees.
- "Constant recruitment for additional faculty has been a part of the work and is discouraging. People come and seem attracted and interest[ed], but we are usually outbid by other agencies offering greater salaries," noted Dean Brocker.

Enrollment:

- 2 full-time freshmen

  * 16 full-time sophomores
  * 5 full-time juniors

- 4 part-time students

Inquiries about the nursing program were received from individuals in 27 North Carolina towns from Pisgah Forest to Wilmington and 10 other states. Four students inquiring about the nursing program at UNC Charlotte noted that they were considering transferring from other schools.

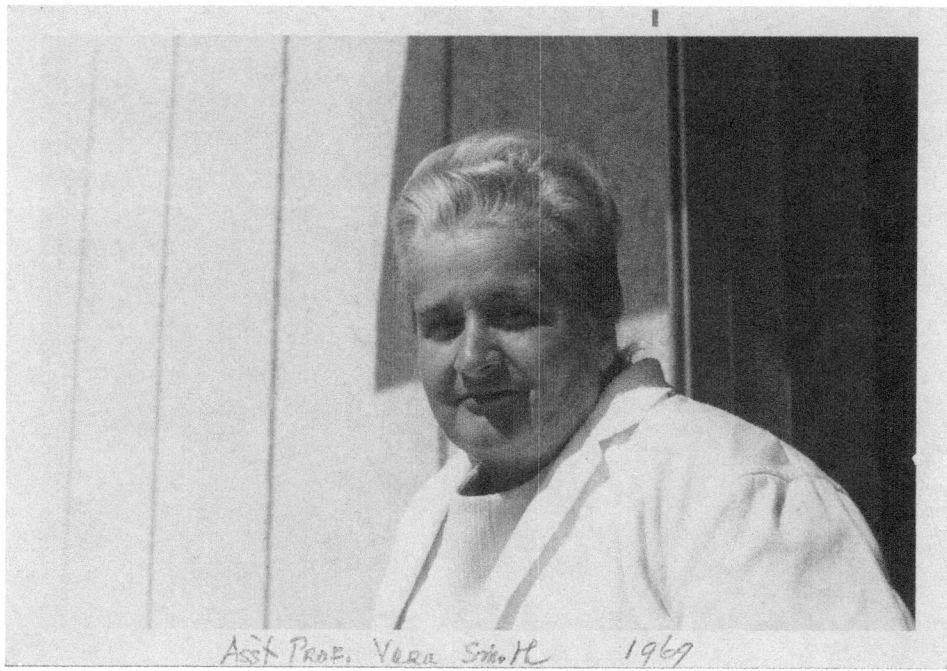

Ass^t Prof. Vera Smith   1969

Vera Smith, third faculty member.

"Key Tasks for the Immediate Future" as noted in Dean Brocker's report include:

- "Since we expect to have four senior students in nursing, we must offer the complete curriculum. This means we must evaluate our program in terms of accreditation criteria and prepare for State Board of Nursing licensure procedures."
- "Establish a plan to offer to RNs as soon as possible."

4th Annual Report of Activities of Nursing
(June 1, 1968–May 31, 1969)[11]

Two additional faculty have been added:

- Professor Joyce Lowder, RN, MSN, now teaches Pediatrics.
- Professor Vera Smith, RN, MSN, teaches Obstetrical Nursing, Mental Health, and Community Health Nursing.
- In April, Instructor Janie Miller, RN, MSN, joined the faculty as a clinical instructor.

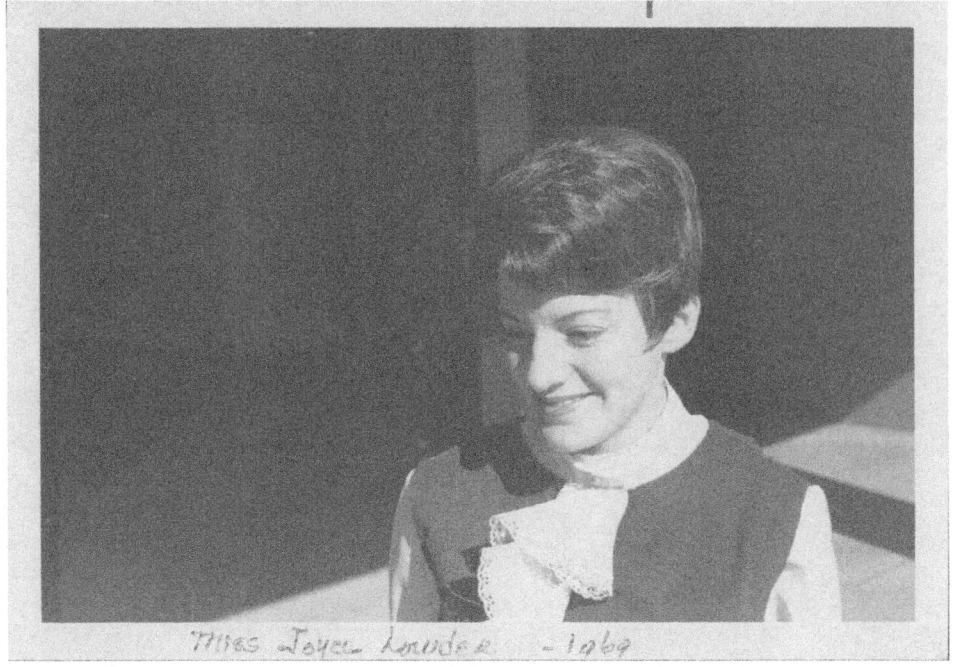

Joyce Lowder, early faculty member.

Highlights of the Major Activities of Nursing

Curriculum:

- Prepared a proposal to modify Fundamentals I and II 201–202 and extend 302, so that more instruction in obstetric and pediatric nursing could be provided.
- Annual reports were compiled and submitted as requested by the National League for Nursing and the NC Board of Nursing.

Faculty-Student Extracurriculars:

- The students requested that Vera Smith, RN, MSN, serve as advisor to their club.
- Joyce Lowder, RN, MSN, attended the Student Nurses' annual convention in Winston Salem with a delegation of UNC Charlotte nursing students.

Recruitment of Students and Faculty:

- No effort has been made to recruit students except to respond to inquiries for information and to participate in Careers for Health Professions workshops.

   * Students of nursing, in uniform, participated in a recruitment program during the annual Festival in the Park.
   * In December, nursing faculty participated in a series of committee meetings to plan campus health facilities.

Other archived data include a copy of a report, dated November 13, 1968, from Tina Green, RN, consultant to Mary McKee, RN, executive director of the North Carolina Board of Nursing. The report was an examination of the nursing program at UNC Charlotte. Excerpts from the findings were:

- Total number of students is 94, as follows:

     * First year   40
     * Second year   21
     * Third year   21
     * Fourth year   12

- Low and high scores achieved on the SAT by students currently enrolled are listed as 717 and 1311, respectively.
- Three students have graduated from this program to date. One of this number performed satisfactorily on the licensing examination.
- The State Board of Nursing visitor understood that university policy allows students to challenge by examination any course offered in the institution. This should prove beneficial to registered nurses who are interested in determining the extent to which previous educational experiences may be applied toward a bachelor's degree.
- "The faculty, as a group, expressed concern related to the distinct improbability that the current number of faculty can effectively implement the nursing courses beginning with the spring semester of 1968–1969. . . . The faculty stated an opinion that a minimum of one additional instructor would be needed to effectively implement the nursing curriculum during the spring semester. The visitor concurs with this opinion." It was noted that plans for the fall of 1969 were to employ one full-time and two part-time instructors.
- In summary, a review of the nursing program and the position it occupies within the organizational framework of the university reflects skillful planning and marvelous potential for strength.

   * The curriculum for the program in nursing appears to be sound.
   * The nursing faculty expressed a remarkable interest in and commitment to the program.

* Students with whom the visitor conversed appeared intelligent, enthusiastic, and highly motivated.
* The program has access to the richest and most abundant clinical resources in the state.
* The major factor threatening the current status and the future growth of this program is the limited number of faculty available to implement the nursing major.
* The urgent need to increase the number of nurses graduating in this state each year was documented recently in a research report, "Nursing Education in North Carolina Today and Tomorrow," published by the North Carolina Board of Higher Education. The necessity of planning for the maximum utilization of both academic and clinical resources for the education of nurses is stressed also in this document. Therefore, it would seem imperative that every consideration be given to providing adequate faculty for this program.
* It is recommended that a minimum of one additional instructor be appointed to nursing effective with the beginning of the spring semester 1969.

The North Carolina Board of Nursing consultant's report[12] was forwarded to Dean Brocker. The report was included in Dean Brocker's annual report to the chancellor with a recommendation for hiring additional faculty. The chancellor, who reports to the president of the UNC General Administration included in his report that he had instituted measures to correct the problem.

Excerpts from the chancellor's Report to the President for 1968–1969[13] references the consultant's report: Chancellor Dean W. Colvard reports that the nursing program was visited by the NC Board of Nursing. Based on the findings, the NC Board of Nursing ruled the institution to be in noncompliance with the requirement for number of faculty and allowed one year to correct the issue leading to the noncompliance. The chancellor noted that two additional faculty members had been appointed for the 1969–70 academic year and a third position was being advertised. He noted, "These additions should accomplish the necessary corrections."

In conversation with Professor Caddell in June 2017, she confirmed that with the addition of the staff as noted in the chancellor's report, full accreditation by the North Carolina Board of Nursing was restored the following year (1970).[14]

Dean Brocker was a visionary. In March 1969, she submitted a communication to Chancellor Dean W. Colvard, PhD, on the subject of a named professorship in nursing.[15] She opens with "Nursing has had a happy a time formalizing some of our special hopes and dreams for our program." She then indicates potential ways in which nursing could utilize "money which you indicated might be available." Some of the ideas that faculty members were interested in exploring were:

- Employing clinical nurse specialists to enrich the program, create partnerships with the hospital, establish an experimental curriculum laboratory for the testing of ideas for content and teaching methods, and developing student-faculty-consultant teams to become involved in social actions for delivery of patient care.[16]
  * Implementing a pilot project in community planning for continuity of care. New modalities of rendering health service to a specific segment of the population could be a means of addressing unmet health needs. Two examples include the geriatric patient and premature infants.[17]
  * Establishing a nurse faculty-student experience in community-service programs. The Southern Regional Education Board Resource Development Project, a consortium of educators promoting educational/community partnerships, could be utilized to provide valuable learning opportunities in an interdisciplinary approach to local and regional problems associated with social and economic changes.[18]
  * Offering a course in a clinical specialty, such as geriatrics.[19]
  * A Seminar on Wheels (a three-week chartered bus trip) to meet national, state, and local leaders involved in nursing and public health programs. For example, the NC State Board of Health, National Communicable Disease Center of Atlanta, medical centers on Indian reservations, National Institutes of Health at Bethesda, and university libraries with special collections of nursing material as a three-hour elective.[20]
  * In order for nursing to attain its proper place in the academic world, faculty who earn the highest degrees in nursing must be employed, and the program needs to be chaired by an individual with a doctorate degree.[21]
- The Dean and Martha Colvard Nursing Distinguished Professorship was established. Dean Edith Brocker's vision became a reality.

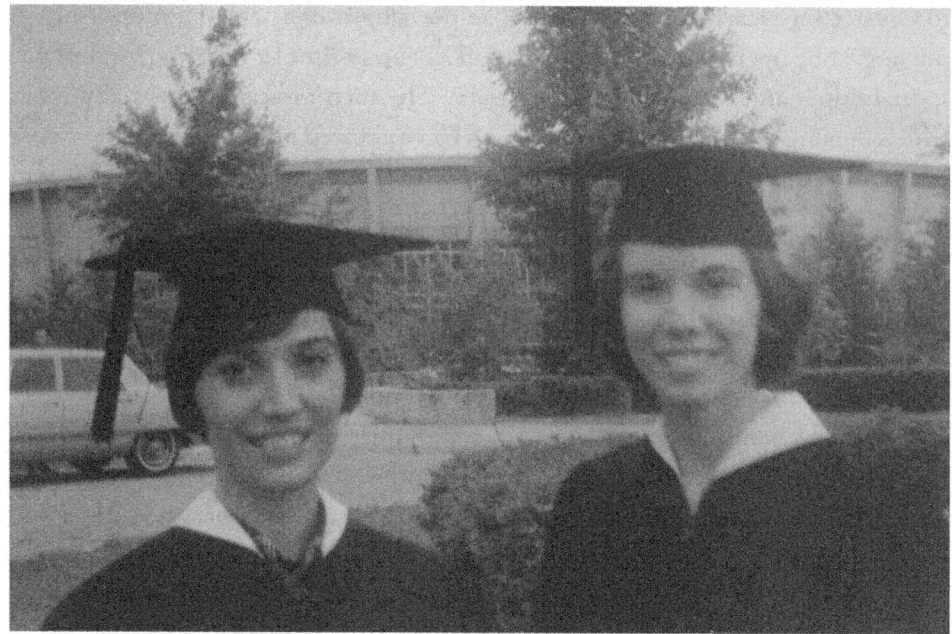

First BSN graduates, Dorothy Alexander and Beth Donnelly.

Student Memories, 1968—1969

BETH DONNELLY, CLASS OF 1968[22]

Prepared by Dona Haney in consultation
with Beth's husband, Terry Alexander

Beth was the second graduate of UNC Charlotte College of Nursing ("Dorothy Alexander was the first," Beth says). Beth started at Charlotte College in 1964. She could live at home, commute for classes, and help take care of her little brother who had Downs Syndrome. She describes that she was meeting with her faculty advisor, "Dr. Heck" and mentioned that she knew she did not want to pursue a degree in biology or to teach. He suggested that she look into "the nursing program, which we are just starting." Beth did and had found her new career path.

Beth began nursing classes with six other students. They were a close-knit group and everything was a first for them and for the school. When her group started clinicals, uniforms were not yet ready. Professor Elinor Caddell, their instructor, described that they wore a white, button-up-the-front uniform that Mr. Smith, the director of nursing at Charlotte Memorial Hospital had located for the students.

Beth remembers several specific patients:

- A little boy who was badly burned. He was about the age of her younger brother. The patient died from infection.
- An adult who was so badly burned, he looked like a skeleton.[23]
- A lady died in the ER from hemorrhage (esophageal varices).
- A terribly injured man who was in his car when he was hit by a train.
- A young man in his 20s who had a traumatic brain injury when the truck tire he was filling with air exploded. He survived, but had lasting issues, so his mother took care of him. He even came to Beth's wedding a few years after he was injured.
- An incident when a doctor had a cardiac arrest on the hospital unit while making rounds. Elinor Caddell went immediately to his side to begin treatment.

Beth shared that when one of her classmates left the program, she sent her uniforms and cap to Beth.

Upon graduation, Beth had a very successful career, largely working in a variety of physician offices. She also was a clinical instructor for CPCC at the OB Clinic and Pediatric Clinic for CMC.

Beth is grateful for her classmates, her college, and her career. She feels fortunate to be in the first class and wishes all the best for the celebration, which she will not be able to attend.

GLORIA JOHNSON, CLASS OF 1970[24]

I was in the first class of the Charlotte College School of Nursing. In my second year, it became UNC Charlotte University and I still remember the bell ringing during the whole day of celebration.

The first year there were six of us in 1965. We were starting our freshman year and the instructors for the nursing school were hired in the second year. I lived at home for my first year, but was so happy to be able to move into the dorms at Memorial Hospital (now CMC) in the second year. Three schools of nursing were in the dorm, the associate, diploma, and BSN. I loved dorm life! We did our clinical at Memorial Hospital, and our courses at UNC Charlotte.

Unfortunately, I did not have a car, but my parents' home was near the campus, and my mother would always fix us lunch before we arrived at UNC Charlotte for classes.

We had most of our meals at Memorial Hospital and were only allowed to wear dresses when entering the hospital.

On my very first day of clinical, I saw a man grab the handrail and sink to the floor. I quickly ran to get my instructor, Elinor Caddell, and she started CPR and saved the life of a physician. She was a hero to me and made me realize the impact a nurse can have on lives.

During this time, the Vietnam War was taking the lives of many young men.

Popular music was Motown, Beach Boys, and the Beatles. The hippy movement was in full swing.

I loved every moment of my 40-year career being a nurse.

SUSAN ALLEN HENDERSON, CLASS OF 1969[25]

Fortunately, I had to work during college to earn money for books and tuition. Working in the UNC Charlotte bookstore between classes allowed me to get to know a lot of the students and professors. Because of their encouragement, I ran for student legislature representative when I was in my first two years in college. My junior year I decided to run for student court and was elected the first female student judge. It was rewarding to be a part of UNC Charlotte's earlier development. You may remember that our school colors started out as light blue before we became "Mean Green." Many decisions were made during those early years. It is an honor to realize we helped set traditions.

Working in the bookstore allowed me to become friends with many of the students from other countries. My family entertained them in our home every Sunday evening and many holidays. Word got out and we soon had students from Queens, Davidson, Central Piedmont, and other area colleges in our home. They shared so much about their countries with us. Many of these students went on to accomplish great things. I am glad to say that many of them still call me "a sister." I live in a very diverse area and those experiences helped me in so many ways.

The summer before my sophomore year, I worked at Presbyterian Hospital and then Charlotte Memorial. That provided me with so many valuable experiences. Many of the nurses would mentor when they knew you were a student. I agreed to work in any area that needed help. Working in such a large hospital gave me so many learning opportunities. I was told that Charlotte Memorial was one of only 10 hospitals in the country doing open-heart surgery at that time. It also showed me a lot of the realities of nursing.

Gary and I married in August 1969. We moved to Oak Ridge, Tennessee. At the time, it was listed as one of the top 10 most educated populaces in the U.S. It also had a very stable work force, yet I was naively optimistic that I would quickly find a job. Those of us who worked at Charlotte Memorial were asked by many unit managers to "Please come back after you graduate." I thought there might be a nursing shortage everywhere. Methodist Medical Center of Oak Ridge (the only hospital in town) had only one job opening in nursing and they really wanted me to take it. I would go to Johns Hopkins and train for six weeks and return as the night manager of the brand new cardiac care unit. That was a great compliment but not appealing to a newlywed.

Soon, though, a wonderful opportunity arrived. They were opening Oak Ridge Mental Health Center, which was a rather new concept for the area. It was a comprehensive care center. Because I had a BSN and just lacked a statistics course [to complete] a second degree in psychology, they hired me to be over the Occupational Therapy Dept. That meant I would be helping develop a program that would include all areas of the center—outpatient and inpatient. It also meant working with patients who had postdoctoral education and a few who could barely read. It was a fun, challenging job that involved lots of creativity and being allowed to think outside of the box, as they say.

I had no family in town and there were no real daycare options at the time in Oak Ridge, so I chose to stay home with our first son, Brock. I never regretted that decision.

After our second son, Michael, was in preschool, I wanted to go back to work part time while they were at school. I went back to the director of the Oak Ridge Mental Health Center and convinced him to let me job-share with another young mother. At the time that was a totally new concept—even to me—but it worked well and they later said that they were glad I had convinced them to try it.

We eventually moved to Knoxville. After our daughter was born, I was very involved with all of the volunteer activities you do when you have three children, so I left nursing for seven years. Fortunately, Park West Hospital near me offered a nursing refresher course and I worked for them after taking the course. Over the 23 years that I worked there, they had various part-time programs, most of which offered "premium pay, but no benefits" and lots of flexibility, which is what I needed. I worked mainly in Psych (which was later called Behavioral Health) and during the last few years, I also worked with the GI Lab. Within Park West Hospital and the large Covenant Health System, I worked mainly on the in-patient unit, but also worked with day programs, clinics, seminars, health screenings, etc. I received my psych. certification through the ANCC. Some weeks I worked as much as 40–60 hours, but generally I worked a part-time schedule. I was able to serve on various process improvement committees, help prepare for Joint Commission, and help to develop some in-patient programs. I also worked in the Education Department and developed a training class for CNAs. The Covenant Health System does not pay more for a BS in nursing, but in some ways they do because they give you more opportunities if you have a BS in nursing. I did find that they were willing to use some of my ideas, including some that dealt with privacy issues long before HIPPA required them to do so.

I am friends with many of the instructors at the University of Tennessee and worked with some of them within the area Psychiatric Nurses Association. They wanted me to go back to graduate school and then teach. By the time the graduate program was really developed at UT, I needed to be earning money for our children's college. Sadly, I found out that hospital pay competes well with what an instructor makes, which is probably why there is such a need for more educators. I did get to do a lot of teaching and mentoring over the years in various ways, which was always fulfilling.

I am now retired but I have organized a very informal group of about 50 (and growing) healthcare workers. We have been meeting for lunch once a month for several years. A lot of positive things have come out of this group. I also try to write letters about healthcare issues to people in Congress. Once a nurse . . .

UNC Charlotte, as we called it, provided many opportunities and taught me that opportunities are always available if we look for them.

NANCY ANN KOHLER RASH, CLASS OF 1969[26]

I entered UNC Charlotte in the fall semester of 1966 as an out-of-state transfer student. I had 53 semester hours completed, but due to illness in May, I was unable to complete the clinical portion of my Nursing Fundamentals II.

I lived in the student dormitory at Charlotte Memorial Hospital with other UNC Charlotte, CPCC, and the final class of CMH nursing students. They all laughed at my New Jersey accent when pronouncing "Howdy, you-all!"

Early that September, Dean Bonnie Cone invited new students, 12 at a time, to her home for an introductory dinner and discussion. I really liked her friendliness and candor. She remembered and called me by name on campus years later. The nursing students helped Miss Caddell design the nursing caps with three scallops at the back, reflecting the six arches at the front of the iconic Kennedy Science Building. Because a black ribbon, denoting a graduate nurse, could not readily be attached to curves, I designed our cap pin, a vertical gold metal bar with UNC Charlotte in gold centered down the forest green enamel. The Division of Nursing (later the College of Nursing) pin also had a scallop arc shape and an oval green stone.

Since I had more credit hours than the usual junior, I consulted Dean Hugh

McEniry to determine whether I could complete another degree concurrently with the BS in nursing. No one had ever gotten a "double degree" or "double major" with nursing. I was close to a BA in psychology, so I took 18 or 15 credit hours and summer classes. Due to the conflict with senior nursing clinical schedules, however, the senior seminar in psychology needed to be taken in the fall of 1969, while I worked 3–11 at CMH in Intensive Care. So I graduated in 1970 also.

While I took summer courses, I worked at CMH Friday and Saturday as a surgical technician on second or third shift. The newborn extended care nursery was especially enjoyable, doing three feedings plus baths 11–7. I was able to "diagnose" a baby who had an inguinal hernia by observing his stooling behavior, cries of pain, bulging scrotum, and his weight gain/loss and feeding and stool records. I told the 7–3 head nurse so she could verify my suspicions and notify the attending resident physician. (She felt he would not recognize a nursing student's finding, but she was "a veteran.") The baby had surgery later that day and recovered completely.

In my operating room experience, I remember the doctor using my right arm as a retractor, and thus letting me feel the "golf ball" surface of a breast cancer tumor that was being excised. I told my future students about that. As a new graduate, Dr. Robicsek asked me specifically to care for his open-heart surgery patients in ICU because he knew I had good training and extra experience with post-operative care.

A happy memory was having a class with breakfast once at Mr. and Mrs. Smith's home, and meeting her husband. They were a warm couple. A sad memory was discovering that a classmate was unable to hear heart and breath sounds when we practiced with our stethoscopes. We met with Dean Brocker and Miss Caddell and my classmate had to switch her major to psychology. (Unfortunately, this was before the day of the American Disability Act and the concept of making adaptations.)

When I was feeling uncertain or stressed, Miss Caddell and Mrs. Smith would help and encourage me. I always wanted to be a good nurse and educator like my mother and like them. I still remember being told, "Your contribution to nursing continues into the future as you teach your students, and also your patients and their families and improve their lives."

Later in my career, I was an infection control co-coordinator, a nursing assistant instructor, and a staff development director at three large nursing homes. I went back to UNC Charlotte and earned my master of science in nursing: nursing education in 1989. While I was teaching associate degree nursing students at CPCC, I was asked to develop a computer-based testing tool to certify nursing assistants. Later I taught this course to the nursing assistants at a nursing center to help them be able to pass the written and the clinical portions of the state test. Some of the older ladies had been working at the nursing center for years. They were happy to learn I could get them through the "scary" parts! State examiners came in to run through the clinical testing and were amazed at how well prepared my students were!

Another example of using my nursing experience in educating happened when I was teaching rescue breathing and basics of CPR one Friday to a first-year CPCC class. On Monday, one student told us that she had stopped her car at the scene of an accident on her way home. She was able to check the victim's pulse (present) and to restart his breathing. The EMTs praised her for her quick work. She told them "Mrs. Rash taught me how to do that in class today!"

I always told my nursing assistant students and my CPCC nursing students that if they got A's and B's from me, they should consider attending UNC Charlotte to get their BS degrees in nursing. It is a great career with a good future.

A happy memory was on May 14, 1969, when a combined wedding shower was held for Barbara Baker and myself at the home of Mrs. Dona Haney. We had a backyard cookout, hand decorated cakes, and presents.

When we took our nursing final exams, Miss Caddell and Mrs. Smith passed us a big bowl of hard candies to share and ease the tension.

We graduated Sunday, June 1st. I married Ronnie Rash on Wednesday, June 4th.

JANET KALE HUNT, CLASS OF 1969[27]

When I graduated from high school in 1965, 12% of men and only 7.4% of women in the United States had completed four or more years of college. At that time, having a college degree was a ticket to upward mobility. My parents were working-class people, and I was the first person in my father's family to attend college.

The establishment of the University of North Carolina at Charlotte that year provided an incredible opportunity to young people interested in earning a bachelor's degree, especially if they lived within commuting distance or were in a position to arrange living quarters near the campus. Best of all, UNC Charlotte was affordable. I had to work part time to pay my way.

I can't remember a time when I was not interested in almost everything concerning medical science. I was also sensitive to human suffering, inequality, and injustice and wanted to understand their causes and do something about them. Even though I had enrolled as a nursing major, I knew deep down that there may be other paths I would follow, and that this degree could give me options.

UNC Charlotte's nursing program was almost brand new in the fall of 1965. I was in the second class of students who would graduate in 1969. Elinor Caddell brought together a few students to design the first uniforms and caps. She was not only an excellent teacher and role model but also a good artist who brought our ideas to life by sketching the designs we suggested. The result, in keeping with university colors, was a forest-green dress with a detachable white apron and a simple white cap.

During the turbulence of the 1960s, it was easy for young Americans to feel unsettled and conflicted, and I was no exception. The country was divided on the key issues of the time: the war in Vietnam, women's equality, and racial discrimination. My family was divided as well.

Once, I was assigned to care for an African American man in the cardiac unit. He was clearly distressed to see a young white woman coming to bathe him, and he said something to me about my not wanting to do this because he was black. I distinctly remember saying, "I'm not like that." He became more at ease, and we proceeded with a comfortable degree of mutual understanding.

During my junior and senior years, I moved from home to live in the former Charlotte Memorial Hospital nursing student dorm. The dorm housed female nursing students from UNC Charlotte as well as students with other hospital-related specialties. We cooked meals in electric popcorn poppers, hung drinks out the window in pillowcases to get them cool, and pierced each other's ears. There is a saying, widely attributed to Alexander Pope, that "a little learning is a dangerous thing." I can't say for sure, but I would bet that every one of us nursing students, at some point or another, diagnosed herself or someone else with the diseases and conditions that were covered in our most recent course of study.

As I look back on the years 1965–69 and my experiences within the College of Nursing, I know that I made the right choice. The education I received was broad enough to reveal a range of future possibilities for work, learning, and new relationships. It was a good start.

Throughout my career I worked in several fields of nursing: medical-surgical, public health, hospice, oncology, and cancer research. My involvement in social and political issues during the 1970s led to foundation-funded jobs in voter registration and public interest research. For a period of time, I wanted to be independent and launched a couple of entrepreneurial endeavors. The most successful enterprise was a wallpaper hanging business. Somewhere in-between I got a second degree in psychology at UNC Charlotte, lived in Germany for five years, and was enrolled as a graduate student in psychology/neuroscience at the University of South Carolina in Columbia.

Finally, it seemed that everything I had done in my life came together to give me all the tools I needed to fit right into a job I could perform with confidence and expertise gained from experience. I spent the last twelve years of my nursing career working in a private oncology practice, and for nine of those years, I worked side by side with Dr. James Boyd, a physician whom I considered to be a master of his craft. This job was the right note on which to end a professional career. I retired in 2014, satisfied that I had, at last, had the best possible job—and that I had given it my best.

LINDA TURNER, CLASS OF 1969[28]

After graduation, nursing provided me with a career for the next 42 years. I was able to help my husband provide for three children and educate all three.

I went back to UNC Charlotte for further education and earned a master's degree in gerontology.

I gained an education for my life, but one of my most special memories from school was my life-long friendship with Anne Sweet. We have been the best of friends our whole lives, always there for each other for the issues life threw at us. We helped each other by building the other one up to get through the difficulties as well as getting in some travel time. I gained a life-long valuable friendship.

Honestly, I am sooooo glad to be retired. I was so tired of nursing at the end. I blame it on aging, but I don't know. From school, the drive was long, and chemistry was so out of this world. Awful. A few classes were fun, but I could not do it again!

DONA HANEY, BSN CLASS OF 1969, MSN CLASS OF 1984[29]

From age four, I planned to be a nurse, probably related to having a young mother who gave up her dream of being a nurse to raise her family, as well as the fact I was the oldest of eight children.

Having spent my growing up years in Charlotte, my family planned that I would go to Presbyterian Hospital School of Nursing. As I began to make plans for graduation, likely the summer prior to my senior year, I obtained information on nursing schools from the NC Board of Nursing and was thrilled to learn that Charlotte College offered a four-year nursing program in which I could live at home. (The real reason: I had then six-year-old brother and sister who I had provided much care for throughout their lives and I was not ready to leave them.) I was accepted into Charlotte College and entered the University of North Carolina at Charlotte. My younger sister says she remembers me bouncing around as I celebrated that I was going to the university rather than a college.

My classmates for the first nursing class, Ecology of Man, taught by Edith Brocker, included freshmen as well as sophomores. We had a great time as a blended course throughout our time of no clinical activity; we heard stories of their clinical experiences and looked forward to our time.

I remember my first patient, a woman with a fracture of the leg. My clinical began at 4 o'clock in the afternoon and this patient agreed to have her bath at that time. It took me three hours to do this bath. Later in my career I would have the opportunity to the clinical instructor for many students having their "first-day-ever" clinical experience. This was always a time of joy and excitement for me as well as those students. In easing their anxieties, I often shared that it took me three hours to bathe my first patient; I think that helped those students begin to understand that everything does not go as we planned it.

One of the things about being in a new program is that new experiences were created for us as well as others. My classmates and I had the opportunity to design the uniforms, caps, and pins; we were also often explaining to people in the hospital how our program was different from the hospital-based programs. After my first year of clinical, I began working as a nurse assistant, so that by my second year of working, I felt prepared to take on additional responsibilities. I approached the staffing person and asked if I could fill a "LPN slot" and do the treatments on a unit for the summer. My request was granted and a new position of surgical technician was created for the new BSN-upperclassmen. I got to work on a single unit for the summer, rather than be rotated throughout the hospital. It was a position that provided more experiences and surely was significant in my comfort level after graduation. It was also a position that would be filled by many others in the years to come.

I chose to work on a medical-surgical unit. After five years, I became the second head nurse appointed who had graduated from UNC Charlotte. Marty Singleton (class of '70) was HN of ICU shortly before my appointment. I later took a position as infection control nurse at Mercy Hospital. This was a new role, a recent JCAHO standard was that all hospitals have an infection control program and a person responsible for coordinating the program. This was a role I thrived in. I have repeatedly thanked Kathryn Gilligan, the person who hired me into this position. One of my unique opportunities was to be a part of the management of the first AIDS patient in Charlotte. I also had the opportunity to become active in the NC Association of Infection Control Practitioners and served as president of this organization for two terms.

I also had the opportunity to enter the first class of the MSN program at UNC Charlotte. My paper in the ethics class centered on some of the issues encountered with the first AIDS patient.

After 30 years in infection control, I fulfilled my high school vision as stated in my graduation booklet: "I will obtain a BA in nursing (at 18 I did not know BS from BA) from Charlotte College (it would become UNC Charlotte that summer) and teach in a university or hospital nursing program." I taught for eight years at the Mercy School of Nursing.

I cannot imagine having a better career than the one I had in nursing. I had numerous opportunities to influence the lives of others with comfort, care, support, and education. I once was with my teaching partner who commented that many of the students saw nursing as a way out of poverty, I responded, "It worked for me!"

I am grateful for the individuals who invested personally in my education and career.

I knew when director of nursing at Charlotte Memorial Hospital Eugene Smith asked me to take a head nurse position and gave me my choice of two units, that Vera Smith had influenced that request.

I continue to count Elinor Caddell as my mentor and very special friend.

BARBARA BAKER MIRGON, CLASS OF 1969[30]

Probably because I had a nurturing mother, I always wanted to pursue a career in nursing. I was attracted to the caring of other people. I had also been exposed to several nurses in my teenage years. I respected them for their knowledge and concern for others.

I chose to attend UNC Charlotte because I was the youngest and only girl in the family. I felt responsible for looking after my parents, who in retrospect were not really old and decrepit (as I had thought at the time) and could have definitely survived with me away at college. Anyway, it was a decision that I never regretted. I also must admit that I was very fortunate because my parents were not overbearing and were supportive. Mom even ironed my uniforms. The things that I didn't have to deal with didn't really slow me down. I learned quickly after I graduated, got married, had children, and went to work. I even learned to cook like Mom.

My memories as a nursing student usually centered around the patients I cared for, the Vietnam War, and the fiancé who became my husband two weeks after graduation. I especially remember a couple of unique moments during Public Health Nursing in our senior year. Being exposed to happenings that I had never experienced in my sheltered life actually helped me grow and not only respect myself, but other people, no matter what the circumstances were. The best memory, however, was belonging to a small class of nursing students who were the first to go through all four years at UNC Charlotte.

Most of my nursing career was in nursing and hospital management. I can certainly attribute my training at UNC Charlotte as preparation for management skills. I began in medical-surgical nursing, but then, after moving to Pennsylvania, I became involved in comprehensive neurological rehabilitation nursing management. Along the way, I was responsible for infection control and development of rehabilitation nursing programs (traumatic brain injury, pain management, and stroke patients). I later became responsible for the quality assurance program in a larger rehabilitation system. While I was there, I developed the utilization management program and was responsible for hospital accreditations and quality improvement, managing the programs of risk management, infection control, utilization management, social work, and medical records. My career involved teaching, program development, and presentations on local and national levels. Realizing that at the time there wasn't anything available on the market for quality assurance in rehabilitation (later quality improvement, quality management, quality systems), I co-authored a book on the subject. Following my desire for always learning, I obtained a master's degree in management with a specialty in healthcare administration.

After spending almost 20 years in Pennsylvania and [putting] our children through college, my husband took a new job in Arkansas. I retired early after the move. I was able to return the favor of my parents' support by caring for my mother in the last years of her life. Now, both being retired, our lives stay pretty full with family, church, and volunteer activities.

KATHLEEN LEDFORD COLLINS, CLASS OF 1969[31]

Prepared by Dona Haney in consultation
with Kathleen's daughter, Robin Collins Taylor

Kathleen and her sister Geraldine started UNC Charlotte in 1965. Geraldine was a history major, but since she was living with her twin sister, she too got to live in the nursing dormitory at Charlotte Memorial Hospital. Kathleen and Geraldine were from South Carolina.

Our classmates were saddened to learn that Kathleen died in 2013 due to complications of diabetes.

Her daughter, Robin, stated that she loved nursing. Her career was in long-term care; she was a nursing home administrator in several locations in Charlotte as well as South Carolina.

She developed gestational diabetes during her last pregnancy and never recovered from it. She was disabled the last 14 years of her life having developed renal failure (requiring dialysis) and blindness.

Her obituary states: "Kathy loved to write short stories and poems. With the help of a computer program, her husband, and her twin sister Geraldine, . . . she had over 100 items published which her family and friends will enjoy and treasure for years to come."[32] Her works include "Through a Woman's Eyes: A Newsletter of Faith," and two poetry books *Purposeful Praise* and *Sowing Season.*

SHELIA FRIEZE NANCE, CLASS OF 1969[33]

Like many of the 1969 graduates, I was the first in my family to attend college. Thanks to my dad's service in WWII, I attended UNC Charlotte on a full Veterans Administration scholarship. Fond memories include Elinor Caddell, instructor. She worked closely with the 12 of us and instilled a sense of pride in our profession. We were so proud of our designs for uniforms, caps, and pins. We were an important part in building a program for ourselves and future nurses. I still have my original cap and pins. Living in the dorm and working as surgical technicians at Charlotte Memorial provided experience and lasting memories. One winter it snowed so deep that I could barely find my VW parked on the side street near the dorm.

One thing that stayed with me all these years is my OR experience. I was in surgery with Dr. Robicsek and scared to death. He took time to have me look closely at the patient's lungs. They were black due to smoking. I never smoked. Throughout my years of practice, I told others what I saw that day in the OR.

I remember the difficulties of my senior year. The Vietnam War was causing the draft of a lot of friends. During that time, Ron got his orders but did not leave right away. He joined the air force and they tried to recruit me due to the need for nurses. We had gotten married the summer following my junior year and were anxious for me to graduate so I could join him. After graduation and boards, we left for Nellis Air Force Base. I had begun work as a graduate nurse at Sunrise Hospital in Las Vegas before learning that I had passed boards and was thankful for the preparation that I had received at UNC Charlotte School of Nursing. It was a happy day when I received notification in the mail that I had passed NC boards. My first RN assignment was staff nurse on a surgical unit. Sunrise was a private hospital serving many entertainers. Elvis was performing there at that time but I never saw him. My first head nurse remains a treasured friend today.

We returned to North Carolina in 1973. I worked part time at Cabarrus Memorial until joining the staff of H&M Medical Clinic. Working with seven internal medicine physicians with specialties in nuclear medicine, cardiology, endocrinology, and respiratory provided me a broad base of knowledge. I served as patient diabetic instructor under the guidance of the endocrinologist. The 12 years at H&M prepared me for my leadership role.

In 1985, I began my career at VAMC in Salisbury. I served as staff nurse for one year before assuming role as nurse manager in geropsychiatry. I earned and maintained certification in geriatric nursing. Providing care for many WWII veterans was my way of giving back to the Veterans Administration and my dad.

Ron retired from the Air National Guard and I from Salisbury VAMC in 2005. Retirement has allowed us time to serve as volunteers, care for aging parents, and help with grandchildren. We continue to enjoy travel with family and friends.

MEMORIES OF RUTH MAULDIN: FACULTY, 1970–1996[34]

I joined the faculty in the fall of 1970 while Edith Brocker was chairman of the then Department of Nursing. Geri Brady and I joined Elinor Caddell, Vera Smith, and Sally Nicholson and we became a full-time faculty of seven. I had known Edith as our assistant dean when I was a student at Duke, and Elinor was a faculty member there when I was a staff nurse and working with the postgraduate recovery room program. It was a privilege to be among persons whom I had held in great esteem a few years previously.

(Joyce Lowder had left that spring before, and JoAnne Norris, Judy Mauldin, and Janie Carlton were already employed.)

When I came for an interview in the spring/summer, nursing had been housed in Garringer building but had since moved into the upstairs of the gymnasium. Edith, Betty Walters, the secretary, and some offices were to the area to the right of the steps while the remainder of the nursing faculty offices were directly across the hall.

I was assigned as coordinator/teacher of Fundamentals of Nursing. Most of our classes were held in the classroom around the corner, which also served as the Nursing Arts Laboratory. The lab held little more than a few beds with bedside tables, two manikins, thermometers, blood pressure cuffs, sphygmomanometers, thermometers, and bandaging supplies.

We used Virginia Henderson's renowned textbook, *The Principles and Practice of Nursing*. Virginia held that "the unique function of the nurse is to assist the individual, sick or well in the performance of those activities contributing to health or its recovery (or to a peaceful death) that he would perform unaided if he had the necessary strength, will or knowledge. And to do this in such a way as to help him gain independence as rapidly as possible."[35] I had high expectations of students. The 1970s was a contentious time in Charlotte politics and our neighborhood in

Myers Park was socially active and demonstrated it with political signs supporting our respective candidates. One morning, my husband woke me telling me that I must come see the newest signs. In front of our house and up the street were signs, "Ruth Mauldin for Governor, She Can Tell You How to Do It!" Along the highway to campus and on the outer door to the gymnasium and the door to the Nursing Department were red, white, and blue signs and decorations with notes saying, "Ruth Mauldin Could Get It Done." Until he left the university, Hutch, the facilities director, called me "Gov" or "Governor."

On another occasion, as I was leaving the office to go home, I found my little white Rambler with gauze dressing around and under with a note saying, "You don't need a procedure book; if you just apply principles, you can remove the dressing." Yes, my students had heard that more than once. I cared deeply that the students would become skilled, knowledgeable, sensitive, caring nurses and thought it was my job to help them to get a good start in that direction. I can say without a doubt that most of them did. It was a joy to teach beginning students and a delight to see them progress so rapidly.

At the end of each year, the nursing division had a picnic in honor of the seniors. These were always an enjoyable occasion for both students and faculty. (I think we had one in 1971 and I believe these were sponsored by the student nurse organization.)

At the end of two years, Mrs. Brocker recommended that I be given permanent tenure. I expressed my displeasure stating that I would have preferred to have been given increased salary instead. Within a few years, I was extremely grateful to have that for some security.

In the spring of 1972, my friend and former classmate at the University of Alabama Nursing School master's program, Dr. Marinell Jernigan, came to visit and while she was there, Elinor Caddell came by to talk with her about the job of dean of the College of Nursing. Soon, Marinell was back for an official interview and was subsequently hired as dean starting in the fall of 1972.

Some of the accomplishments or happenings during her tenure as dean include:

- A group of students went to the Sloan Kettering Hospital in New York to learn about nursing practices there during the time that the UNC Charlotte basketball team was playing in the semifinal game of the NIT.
- A group of students went to London to the Florence Nightingale School.
- The consortium between UNC Charlotte and UNC started the master of nursing program.
- The program achieved NLN accreditation in December 1974.

- All of the preliminary groundwork was done for the establishment of the Gamma Iota Chapter of Sigma Theta Tau, which was chartered in 1978.

In the mid-1970s I was assigned to teach and coordinate critical care. At various times, Patty Gray, Jean Campbell, Delores Sanders, Lynn Coleman, and I taught the class content and had various part-time faculty helping with clinical supervision. This was much more in keeping with my style and temperament. Critical care was a seven-week course and when we began, we had students rotating through coronary care, intensive care, and emergency care for clinical experience. The students were spending so much time getting oriented to the new clinical setting that Jean Campbell, Pat Yaros, and I developed a series of slide tape programs to orient students to the various areas and to teach some of the content. One of our programs was accepted for presentation at an AV Fair in New Jersey. Jean Campbell and I were excited to go and present our program.

There was some discord beginning within the faculty and cliques were developing despite the progress of the college and the success of the students.

Dr. Jernigan retired effective in the fall of 1977.

I was appointed to the search committee and we reviewed several candidates and brought three to the university for interviews. The last one to be interviewed was Louise Schlachter. Several members of the committee were extremely impressed with her vitae and her presentation. Jean Crawford and I expressed some concern regarding, among other things, her statements about how she would handle dissenters. I felt that perhaps I had a biased view and hoped that she would indeed bring cohesion to the faculty.

However, on her first day in the office, a Monday, Dr. Schlachter had flowers on her desk and said these had been delivered to her house on Friday from her faculty at Pace wishing her good luck and telling her how they had missed her. The flowers were beautiful, in perfect condition, and one could easily imagine the drops of dew from their recent removal from a floral refrigerator. Flowers seemed to follow her. She once received a large bouquet of flowers at the chancellor's house when he was having a faculty party.

Dr. Schlachter almost immediately began driving wedges between faculty members, telling some of vicious acts that others were doing to her. She rewarded some with gifts, invitations to her home, and trips to professional meetings while others were negated. During her tenure, I was never given more than the minimal raise and upon her departure, my salary was almost doubled (due in part to an elevated position and to working for part of the summer to help get ready for the fall).

One Friday evening when I had students working in the emergency room, one of the security policeman asked me if I knew that "crazy lady" who was "head of nursing at UNCC." He knew about her because he had been involved when she called to report a snake "that one of her faculty had placed in her mailbox." At another time, he said that she had reported that her shrubs had been torn out of the ground.

During this period of time, I taught Critical Care Nursing. It is an area that I am especially fond of and my teaching, especially clinical supervision of students, was extremely rewarding. The students were senior level and often experienced those "ah-ha" moments when things come together. At such times, faculty are often given credit when in actuality the student has synthesized knowledge that has been gained over time. It gave one a good feeling about what the curriculum had helped the students achieve.

However when a student fails a course, especially at this level, it is extremely difficult both for the faculty and the student. One of my highlights of teaching was to get a Christmas card from a student who had failed her last course, Critical Care, and had to come back the following fall to repeat it. The card, sent a year later, stated that Critical Care had helped her to gain a degree of self-confidence that she had never had before and she wanted me to know how it had helped her.

Those types of experiences, along with the faculty that I worked with, was what kept me at the university. Jean Campbell, who had been one of the faculty in Critical Care had resigned at the end of the first semester after Dr. Schlachter came. Lynn Coleman, Dee Sanders, Patty Gray, and I worked very amicably. Lynn and I wrote an article "Intracerebral Herniation" and had it accepted for publication in the *Journal of Neurological and Neurosurgical Nursing* in 1985.

Rumor had it that there was increased security around the speaker's platform at graduation in 1984 and on the following day, the faculty were called together and told that Dr. Schlachter had been relieved from her position as dean. Coming with tenure, she could not be fired without a lawsuit and that would have been more damning to the university and the college.

Pauline Mayo was elected by the nursing faculty to serve as acting dean for a year. We were implementing a new curriculum and there was much to be done. I was elected Area Head of Level 3, which was the senior year. Dr. Schlachter was given the fall semester off and was assigned in the spring as a faculty member in Level 3. Students had to write a paper, which counted as a part of their overall grade and clinical performance also counted a part of their total grade. She gave all of her students an excessively high grade on their papers and an A in their clinical performance. The area faculty decided that if any clinical instructor gave unusually high grades on their papers, that a second faculty would be asked to grade papers as well. Dr. Schlachter wrote a letter to the university lawyer complaining about me for having "interfered with her academic freedom." She threatened to sue both the university and me. The lawyer responded that the action was taken by the entire faculty in the area and that any other faculty member would be treated likewise.

A search committee was established and was successful in bringing Nancy Langston to the college in 1985.

We implemented a new curriculum in 1997 and I coordinated "Adult Health I."

I took a leave of absence 1990 to 1991 and when I returned I became coordinator of the beginning course in nursing and coordinator/director of the Nursing Laboratory in the Colvard Building.

Sue Bishop had become the dean of the College, which had become the College of Nursing and Health Professions.

I retired in 1996.

Leah Foster (now Smith) graduated in 1995 or '96. She was the first nursing student to graduate from the University Honors Program and received several awards that year. I have asked her to submit some memories. She was an excellent student!

JOYCE ANN LOWDER[36]

On being a UNC Charlotte CON faculty member 50 years ago

I am Joyce Ann Lowder and I joined the faculty immediately after graduation from Emory University with a master's degree in nursing (MSN), which covered the areas of obstetrics and pediatrics; my subspecialty was pediatrics.

I was the youngest ("greenest") member to join the faculty; there were three others at that time: Dr. Edith Brocker, Elinor Caddell, and Vera Smith. I recall feeling intimidated being the "youngest one on the block," but I was immediately admitted into the faculty family. My only teaching experience had been in a diploma program for about a year.

My wish was to help the students to develop their hopes and dreams of becoming the best nurse possible. I wanted them to continue their desire for education following their graduation from UNC Charlotte CON. I also wanted to convey the importance of being physically, emotionally, and spiritually strong in their professional nursing roles. I felt privileged to

have their trust and the trust of their parents/loved ones as they had invested their hopes, support, and resources to see the students succeed. I was so proud of the students! They looked professional in their green and white uniforms, but they wore compassion and courage in their hearts as they faced each new challenge! UNC Charlotte added to their courage!

I apologize for being unable to recall the students, so long ago. I do recall one student, now Lynn Dobson, who was a leader, as I recall, in the Student Nurse Fellowship. She was energetic and humorous; there was mischief lurking in her smile. However, she was an excellent student and has continued to be a leader in her profession and family and church life.

I have very fond memories of Dr. Edith Brocker, from my first interview with her. Her gentle spirit, coupled with high expectations for the growth of the program, were most impressive and appreciated! She had dreams of the success of this program. She worked incessantly; not easy, when the nursing program was small, compared to other departments. I respected her so much that I decided to stitch a pair of lace gloves for her. I finished them, late at night, before the Christmas party the next day. I placed them out to look at them . . . and found that I had made two right-hand gloves!!!! Yes, I did take out the stitches and fixed the problem, on time!

I also must acknowledge my role model on the faculty: Elinor Caddell. We must have looked like Mutt and Jeff, as she was tall and I was, well, petite. She was tall in more ways than stature! She shared her knowledge, compassion, encouragement, and expertise with me at a time when I really needed it. Her wisdom, common sense, and professionalism was a blessing! There were times when we needed lunch and she would invite me to join her, and her dear mother, on the front porch for a bologna and pickle sandwich after we had completed a clinical morning. She will always hold a special place in my heart! She has had an unforgettable impact on nursing, UNC C CON, students, patients, and me!

Vera Smith was also someone who helped me, especially when I had no experience in the clinical setting of Charlotte Memorial Hospital. My home base of experience had been Presbyterian Hospital School of Nursing. Vera was very knowledgeable, knew everyone, and had a warm heart!

I left UNC Charlotte CON three years after being on the faculty. My goal was to deepen my knowledge in pediatrics, so I expected that it would take about two years, and then I hoped to return. I went to Omaha, Nebraska, where there was a children's hospital, and I joined the University of Nebraska College of Nursing. The two years became 20 years, and my experience in pediatrics was deepened, along with so many other learning opportunities.

I believe that UNC Charlotte CON was the springboard for my teaching experience in Nebraska. I am forever grateful for this springboard and I am so glad to see that it has grown by leaps and bounds! I applaud your efforts in trying to gather the ramblings from me and others. I must say that the memory is nowhere near what I wish it was, but I am grateful for all that God has allowed me to see and do.

Class Pictures of Classes 1968–1971

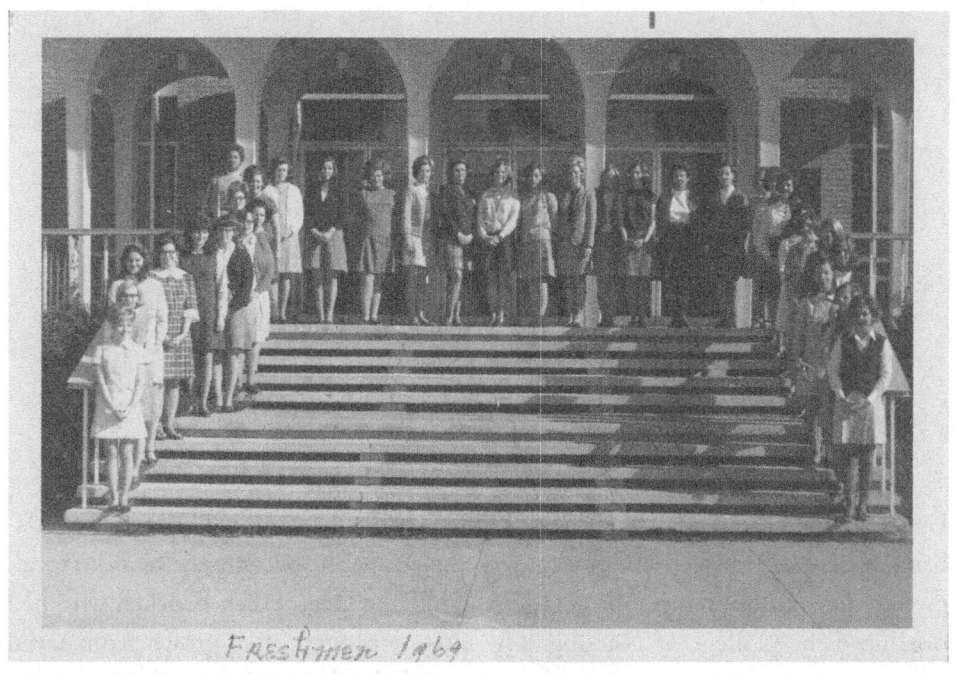

Freshmen 1969

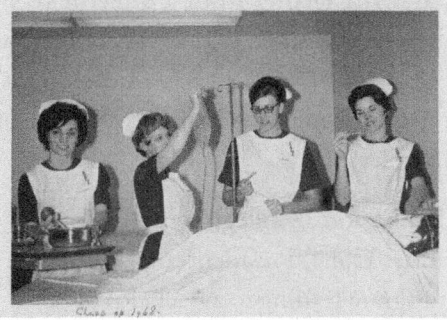

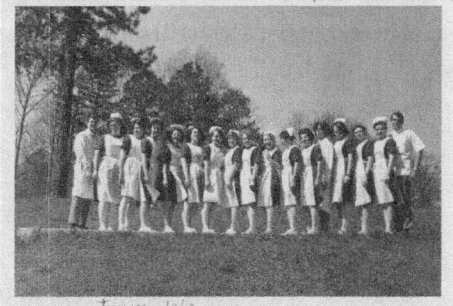

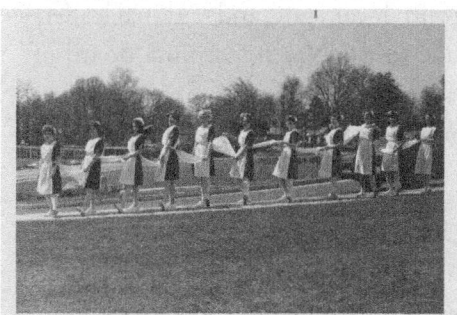

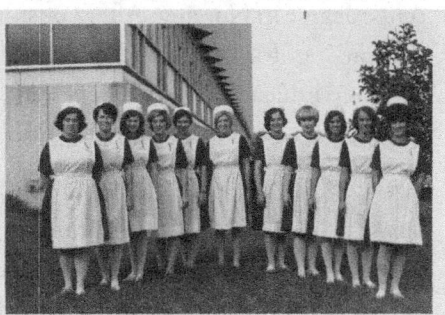

Classes 1969–1972.

CHAPTER TWO

Rapid Growth and Development

Dr. Marinell Jernigan, 1972–1977

Ann Mabe Newman, RN, PhD

Dean Marinell Jernigan, RN, came to UNC Charlotte from the University of Alabama, where she earned her doctorate in education. She became the first doctoral-prepared dean of nursing and replaced the retiring Dean Edith Brocker, who had organized the College of Nursing. The nursing program had grown from seven students in 1965 to 260 students by 1973, and the faculty from a director to 13 faculty members. Dr. Jernigan's tenure can best be described as one of exponential growth and development.

Dr. Jernigan begins her annual report (1972–73)[1] with a historical overview of nursing's role in the development of the university:

> In the spring of 1963—the year in which Charlotte College evolved from a two-year to a four-year institution—Bonnie Cone, President and founder, gauged interest in the establishment of a program leading to a Bachelor of Science degree in Nursing. After consulting with local, state, and national leaders in nursing, formal consultation was made to the North Carolina Board of Higher Education. Upon receiving a favorable response, an application to "establish a School of Nursing" was submitted to the NC Board of Nursing Registration and Nursing Education on May 18, 1964.

> Permission for a School of Nursing at UNC Charlotte was granted, and in the spring of 1965 the program began with seven students and a director. The following year, the program had expanded to include a faculty member and a total of 52 students. Ensuing years were crowded with the activities of seeking qualified nursing faculty, developing curriculum, designing the student uniform and school pin, and

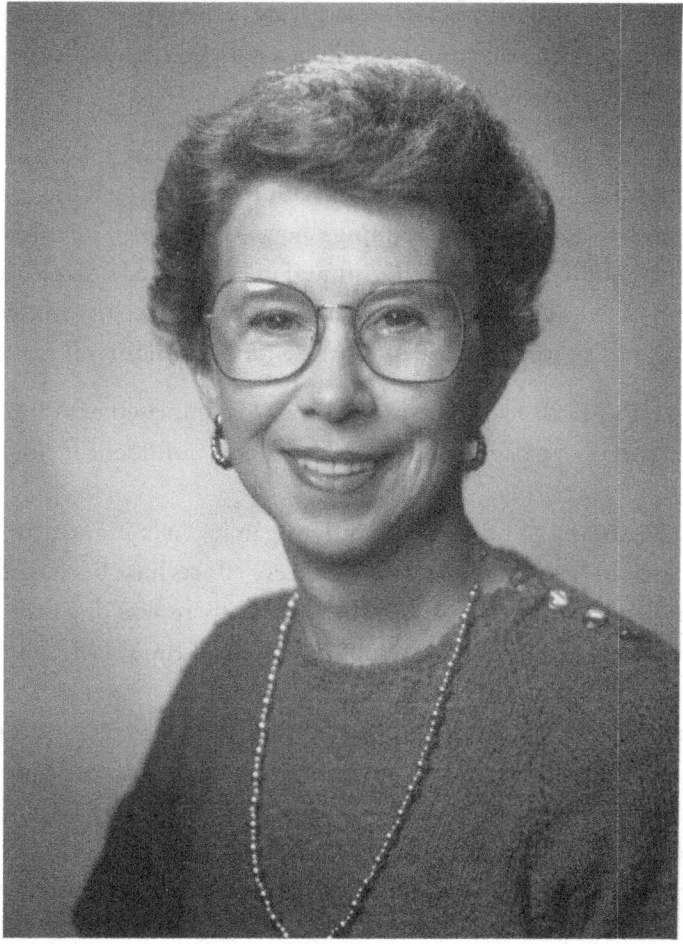

Dr. Marinell Jernigan.

three changes of address. In 1968, the fledgling nursing program graduated its first class of three, two in May and one in December.

Begun as a department in Charlotte College, nursing became a division in the new university structure, and on November 13, 1970, was renamed the College of Nursing. The student population increased each year along with the nurse faculty. Currently, the full-time teaching faculty numbers 13 with a student body of approximately 270. This growth in numbers of nursing students brought an ever-increasing demand for more clinical facilities for learning experiences. The clinical agencies in which nursing students now practice include a local 900-bed hospital as well as other specialty facilities—rehabilitation hospital, nursing center, county health departments, selected physician's offices, and clinics.[2]

Capturing the spirit of the faculty at large, and especially the nursing faculty as they worked during the early years of making a college, required time and energy. The 1973–74 university catalog stated:

> A team of outstanding educators has been assembled to give leadership to a young and highly qualified faculty. Faculty members at UNC Charlotte have accepted the challenge of building a new institution. They are willing to sacrifice the stability they might have found in established universities for the satisfaction of helping to build a new and modern university, which is aware of and receptive to its commitment to the wider community it serves.[3]

In 1971–72, the College of Nursing faculty was comprised of 11 full-time members. The year 1972–73 began with an experienced, confident faculty and a new dean.

From the beginning of her tenure, Dr. Jernigan had a commitment to ensuring faculty diversity. In her report she states, "Sincere efforts have been made to recruit nurse faculty among minority groups. In the fall, there was one full-time faculty member who was black. The college employed two full-time black faculty members in the spring term."[4]

Approximately half the students enrolled in the College of Nursing resided in the dorms, while half lived off-campus and commuted daily. Student enrollment began to rise quickly with 77 freshmen, 76 sophomores, 72 juniors, and 40 seniors for a total of 265 undergraduate students. Two representatives from each of the three upper levels worked with faculty throughout 1972 to review and evaluate the curriculum.

Nursing students were members of the three social sororities on campus, and a nursing major was chosen "Miss 49er" for the 1972–73 school year. The college had representation on the University Forum Committee, and a junior nursing major was elected by the university as associate justice on the university court. The Student Nurses' Association, the professional organization of nursing students, met monthly with an average attendance of 25–30 students. Faculty actively supported this group. While there were no significant changes in the curriculum during that academic year, students were involved with faculty throughout the year in systematic evaluation of the curriculum in preparation for seeking national accreditation. The accreditation visit by the National League for Nursing was scheduled for early fall 1973, and in 1974, accreditation was granted.

In his letter of congratulations, Chancellor D. W. Colvard wrote: "Dear Dr. Jernigan, on behalf of the entire university, I wish to extend to you and the faculty of the College of Nursing our sincere congratulations on having your program ac-

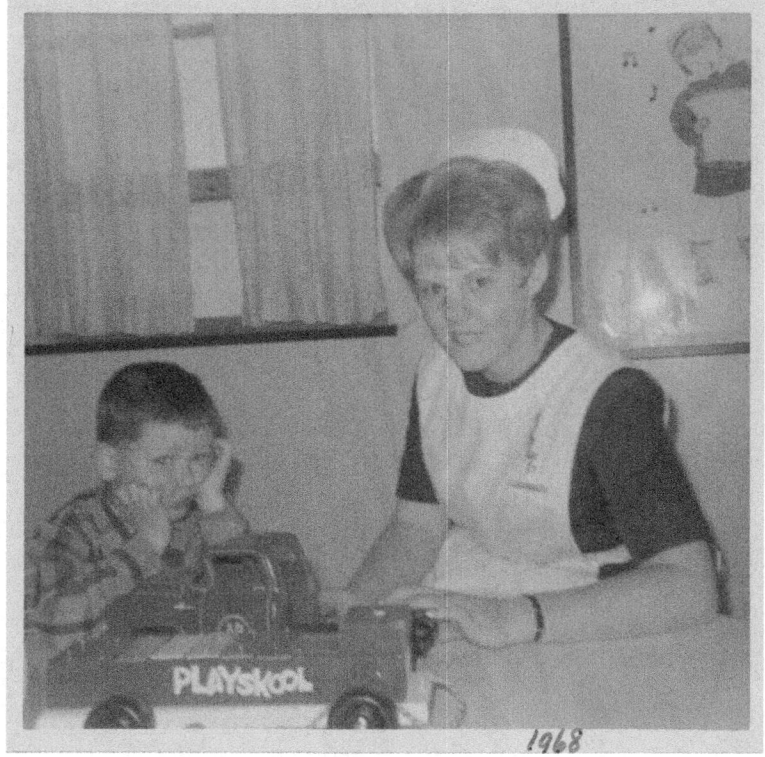

Pediatric clinical, 1968.

credited by the National League for Nursing. This achievement continues to reinforce the fact that we are developing an excellent program in Nursing."[5]

Letters from across the university recognized this as a milestone. Dr. Newton Barnette from engineering wrote: "Having gone through a similar process, we in engineering know what a great undertaking the building of an accreditable program is and how rigorous the visitation preparation is."[6]

In addition, there was this touching handwritten note from our founder Miss Bonnie: "I rejoice in the good news of the accreditation of our Nursing program by the NLN. Bravo for you and your teammates! Sincerely, Bonnie E. Cone"[7]

In her 1974–75 annual report, Dr. Jernigan listed many of the significant achievements and accomplishments of the year. At the top of the list was "NLN Accreditation, 1974." Another important milestone: "Modification of uniform dress and adoption of pantsuit."[8] Tasks accomplished that may seem mundane now but were vitally important in the building of a new college included: application for federal construction grants with very significant faculty input, application for capitation funds, designing and printing of new nursing brochures, and pro-

The University
of North Carolina
at Charlotte
UNCC Station
Charlotte, N. C.   Office of
28223   the Chancellor

                                                         704/597-2201

                                    December 12, 1974

        Dean Marinell Jernigan
        College of Nursing
        UNCC

        Dear Dean Jernigan:

        On behalf of the entire University, I wish to extend to you and
        the faculty of the College of Nursing our sincere congratulations
        on having your program accredited by the National League for
        Nursing, Inc. This achievement continues to reinforce the fact
        that we are developing an excellent program in Nursing.

        Please convey my congratulations to the faculty for their role
        was instrumental in attaining this accreditation.

        With kind regards, I am

                                        Sincerely yours,

                                        D. W. Colvard
                                        Chancellor

        DWC/ew

        cc: Dr. Frank Dickey
             Dr. Philip Hildreth

Note of congratulations from Dr. Colvard on NLN accreditation, 1974.

cedures for faculty evaluation adopted for a two-year trial period. Even though she was helping to build a new college, Dr. Jernigan realized the importance of reviewing the process periodically to ensure it was working.

The interaction of faculty and students was important and duly noted in the report: "Student/faculty Halloween party, Van Landingham House; faculty committee: Norris, Mauldin, Harvey, Brady, and Mobley." Staff were also an important part of the team. Dr. Jernigan noted, "Success in gaining new staff position—even more successful in filling it—Peggy Overcash."[9]

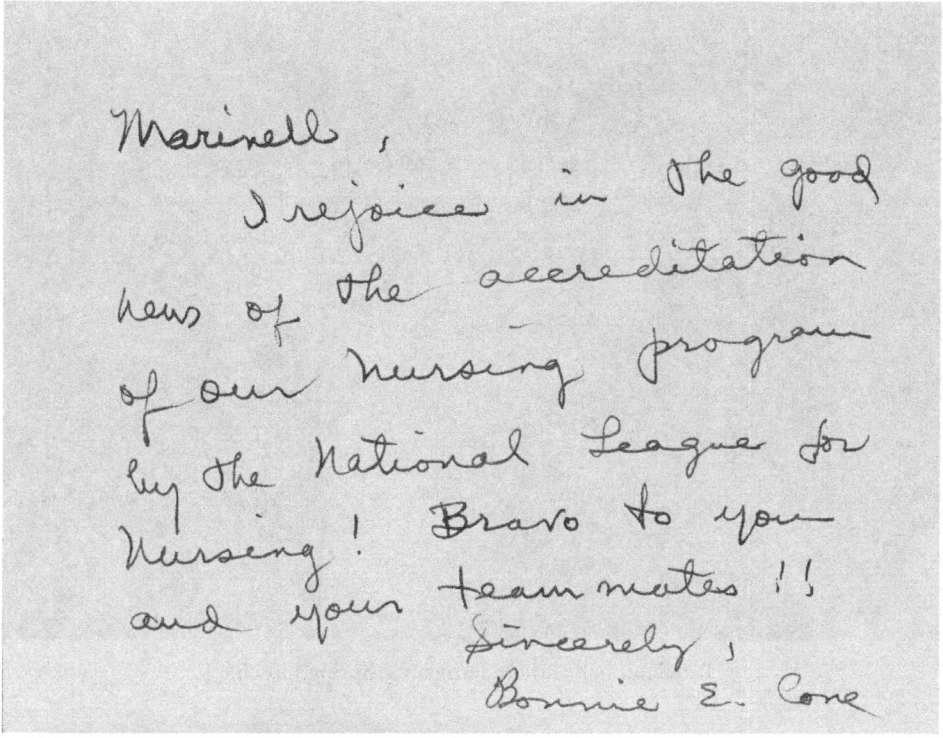

Handwritten note of congratulations from Bonnie Cone on NLN accreditation, 1974.

In her summary, Dr. Jernigan was already looking to the future. With NLN accreditation complete, she noted that following the achievement of this goal, "recruitment of qualified faculty to assist with the development of a graduate program leading to a Master of Science in Nursing degree assumes a high priority."[10]

Reports can only tell us the facts. Moreover, the facts of Dr. Jernigan's tenure reveal her many accomplishments, and there were many. The unique memories that flow from an oral history reveal the philosophy, experience, and excitement for the topic. In June 2017, I had the delightful opportunity to spend time talking to Dr. Marinell Jernigan at her home.[11] The ambiance, the setting, and the hospitality of the visit set the stage: Upon my arrival, I was met by the exquisitely dressed but casual, petite woman, with the funkiest red-framed eyeglasses you have ever seen, Dr. Jernigan. After years of knowing her I still am not comfortable calling her Marinell. We had Bloody Marys in her beautifully decorated living room and began our conversation, adjourning only for lunch.

We talked about her life postretirement from UNC Charlotte: She remarried at 65 and says "these have been the greatest 20 years of my life." Their love story

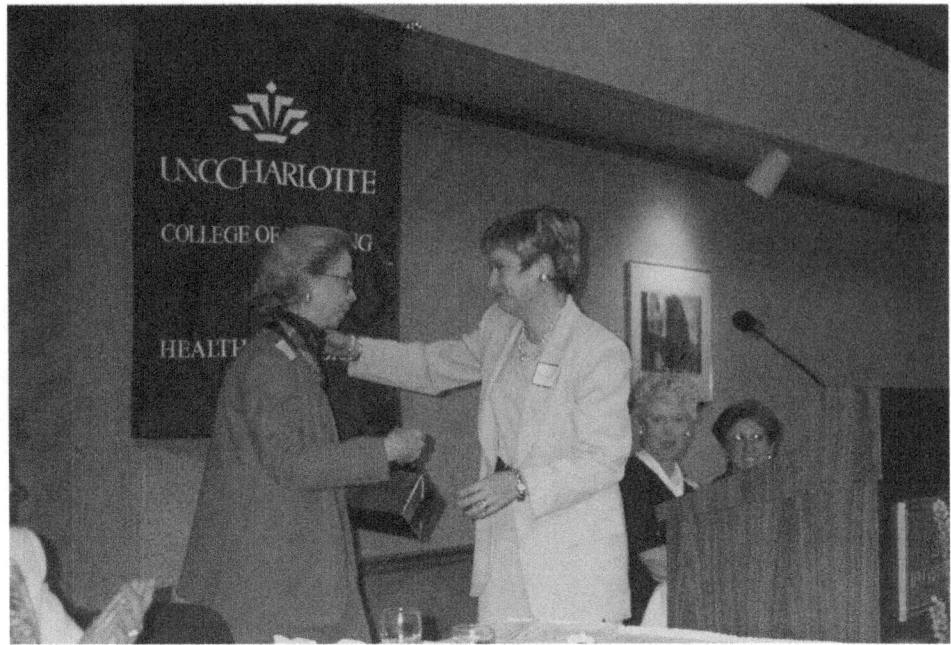

Pat Campbell and Dr. Jernigan at Spring Lunch.

was heart-warming. She and her husband have traveled extensively and their fitness routines put most of us to shame!

I had a list of questions and remarks from her reports that I wanted her to expand on. Three hours later, I had my answers:

AMN: You and your faculty were certainly ahead of your time in declaring "health care is a right."

Dr. J: Well remember that we were writing our first self-study and we had never before been asked to put on paper what we believed. The faculty worked very hard to define the role of nursing in helping people obtain optimal health.

AMN: In the self-study, you wrote: "We believe that nursing is an important social force which makes an essential contribution to the total health of society. We further define professional nursing practice as being deliberative, interactive, scientifically based and devoted to helping individuals, families, and groups make maximum use of their internal and environmental resources in meeting their respective health needs." How did you and the faculty go about designing a curriculum to attain these goals?

Dr. J: The program was over five years old when this self-study was done. The curriculum was pretty standard for BSN programs, but we refined it and made it unique to our students and our beliefs. We had an experienced faculty who had taught in other programs across the nation and their input helped to shape our curriculum.

AMN: During the early days of the program about 90% of senior nursing students lived off campus. Where did they live?

Dr. J: Most lived at home, but through 1973 housing was available for a limited number of nursing students in the residence halls at Charlotte Memorial Hospital. In the summer of 1973 the fourth high-rise dorm housing 500 students was completed bringing total campus housing to 2,000. So many nursing students moved to campus in the fall of 1973. There were two cafeterias on campus—one adjacent to the dorms for those students living on campus and one located in the Cone Center used by commuting students, faculty, and staff. It was necessary at times for the CON to negotiate with cafeteria management for early breakfasts for students having morning clinical experiences at the hospitals.

AMN: And the bookstore was in the Atkins Library and the nursing lab was in the Student Health Center?

Dr. J: Yes and our faculty offices were in the Health and Physical Education Building and shared with the Department of Health and Physical Education. And with classes taught across campus, some days it was like a marathon to make the rounds. So, you can imagine my disappointment when our proposal for building space for the CON was turned down by the Legislature. The proposal for the building was later submitted and funded.

AMN: Macy, Rowe, Winningham, Denny . . . these were some of the first buildings on campus. Did nursing hold classes there?

Dr. J: Yes, we used all of those buildings. And for clinical space in addition to Charlotte Memorial Hospital, we utilized Charlotte Rehabilitation Hospital, Charlotte Eye, Ear, Nose, and Throat Hospital, Wesley Nursing Center, Mecklenburg Health Department, Randolph Clinic, and Mecklenburg Mental Health Center. We were growing so fast that contracts with all of these agencies became an almost overwhelming task.

AMN: The number of faculty grew exponentially also. You began your tenure as dean with 13. How many were there in 1977 by the end of your tenure.

Dr. J: There were 26, so yes, as we enrolled more students, we needed more qualified faculty and classrooms and clinical space. The College of Nursing was thriving and we were very proud of the contributions we were making to the university and the community.

AMN: Since you hired all of these faculty, I thought it might be nice to name these early movers and shakers who helped build all of the programs: E. Caddell, M. Jernigan, P. Haynes-Mayo, E. Leonard, S. Nicholson, V. Smith, M. Anderson, A. Cahill, J. Campbell, K. Chitty, S. Cox, S. Harvey, R. Mauldin, C. Maynard, C. Mobley, S. Morgan, J. Norris, P. Sykes, P. Yaros, G. Davenport-Cook, S. Doyle, N. Gentry, P. Lawrence, D. Sanders, C. Stitt, and L. Whitlock.

Dr. J: Two staff support people were also very important to the success of the college: Betty Walter and Peggy Overcash. Many of these dedicated faculty members stayed with us until retirement and helped build the graduate program during my tenure.

AMN: One of the annual reports sent to you, written by Elinor Caddell, was regarding the Outreach Graduate Program at UNC Charlotte and UNC Chapel Hill. I'll cite part of the report and ask you to comment on it:

> During 1973 and early 1974 Deans of the Schools of Nursing in North Carolina were most eager to have graduate level offerings at their universities [and] met a number of times in an advisory capacity to formulate plans for such a project. Interest by the Deans and the Graduate Faculty of the School of Nursing at Chapel Hill was generated by the constant pressure from nurses throughout the state for graduate education in nursing that would be readily available to them. Naturally nurses most affected by a geographical extension of our program are those whose families are well established in communities a considerable distance from Chapel Hill making it difficult to impossible for entering the program at Chapel Hill.

In April 1974, following a thorough review of the George and Booth study, and following exploratory discussions with Vice Chancellor Sheps and Dean Lyle Jones, the graduate faculty recommended to Dean Lucy Conant that the first outreach program site should be located at UNC Charlotte. This decision was based on the number of potential students in the area, availability of excellent clinical facilities, the potential pool of faculty and preceptors in Charlotte, and that Charlotte had its own AHEC. Dean Conant contacted Dean Jernigan, who gave the project her blessing. Dr. Jernigan received both approval and enthusiastic support for the program from university administration.

Early in May, representatives from UNC-Chapel Hill School of Nursing and from the UNC Charlotte College of Nursing met for preliminary discussions and planning. Professor Elinor Caddell was designated the Director of the Outreach Graduate Program in Charlotte. Planning between the schools continued on a weekly basis, primarily between Betty Sue Johnson, Director of the Graduate Program, UNC Chapel Hill, Elinor Caddell, Director of Outreach Graduate Program, and the Medical-Surgical Nursing graduate faculty at Chapel Hill.

In 1973, UNC-Charlotte College of Nursing's five students began their first year of the master's program. They, with the Outreach Director, made a weekly trip to Chapel Hill to participate in course work with the students in the Medical-Surgical Nursing major at UNC-Chapel Hill SON. The first year went well, and we are planning to admit six students from the Charlotte area into the program next year.[12]

Dr. J: This project gave evidence of the College of Nursing's growing influence on nursing in North Carolina. Because of its success, we were able to make an easy case for our own master's program a few years later.

AMN: In summarizing the strengths of the College of Nursing in the National League for Nursing Self-Study you stated: "The college is comprised of a faculty group who work well together, disagree agreeably, are not afraid to try new ideas and approaches, and who are not afraid to fail." This is a remarkable statement. Tell me more.

Dr. J: The late '60s and early '70s were years of growth and change in the profession. We were a part of that growth. We had a committed faculty. Hospital nursing care was changing to include more home and outpatient care. This change had a great impact on our curriculum and trying new ideas and approaches was necessary. Conflict was a natural part of that and the faculty had to feel safe and supported. Disagreeing agreeably became our strength. We were a strong faculty and as such we were able to move nursing education to a new level of success.

Student Memories, 1970s

ANN MABE NEWMAN, RN, PHD, CLASS OF 1978, FACULTY, 1980–2012[13]

My initial encounter [as a student] with the College of Nursing was less than positive. I had been an RN for twelve years when I applied to the UNC Charlotte program. We had moved to Charlotte in 1968 having barely escaped Vietnam. I heard about a new nursing program at UNC Charlotte. My kids were in kindergarten and I was finally ready to pursue my BSN. I was essentially told that I would have to earn 120 hours like all other beginning students. No credit for my diploma in nursing from The University of Virginia. I did not take it well. I "pouted" for almost a year before I figured out how to take advantage of the challenge system. Betty Walters the secretary in the CON encouraged me to contact other RN's who were in the program. We formed a support group called the "PRN's." I had the opportunity to be a student representative on the new Pathways program for RN's returning to get a BSN and the rest is history.

I fell in love with learning again. I was a charter member of Gamma Iota of Sigma Theta Tau. I met innovative professors like Eleanor Leonard who let me design my own clinical for the management classes, and I was turned on to teaching by observing the enthusiasm of a new professor, Glenna Davenport-Cook. I went to New York with a group of students led by Betsy McClain to see state-of-the-art rehabilitation at Montefiore Hospital in Brooklyn. I must admit that my favorite part of the trip was seeing Yul Brynner in *The King and I.* I was briefly able to convince my classmates that the gold earring Yul Brynner was wearing was my missing one.

JoAnne Norris my advisor was always so supportive. She suggested an elective that had a great impact on my career, called Women and Politics taught by Dr. Patricia Kyle. At a District 5 NCNA meeting which students were required to attend, I had an "a-ha" moment when I realized the potential for nurses to affect and improve patient care through participation in the political process. I also made the decision to always sign my name "RN" as a way of letting people know not only how proud I am to be a nurse but because it was a way to influence the political process.

The friends, colleagues, professors, and insights I gained as a student at UNC Charlotte's College of Nursing affirms my notion that I was nurtured by the best.

Another RN completing her BSN, Gerry Roberts, influenced me to go to graduate school. Long before we had our own graduate program at UNC Charlotte, pioneers like Elinor Caddell and Dean Marinell Jernigan began a graduate program with Chapel Hill for RN's in the Charlotte area. I and five other RN's went to Chapel Hill once a week and had class with the students there. Elinor Caddell supervised our clinical experiences in Charlotte. With no cell phones, no computers to rely on, the five of us took turns going to the Greyhound Bus Station to pick up a tape recording of the seminar we were expected to discuss the next day. Lynn Coleman and Angel Vasquez and I did our thesis project together at CMC looking at the effect of noise on pain in the recovery room. We were thrilled when an abstract was published in the *American Journal of Nursing.* Lynn Coleman and I went on to become faculty at UNC Charlotte. Lynn and I have remained friends over the years since we graduated in 1980.

By now I am starting to bleed green and the hemorrhage has continued. I taught for 34 years and am now an active nursing alumni and chair of the UNC Charlotte retired faculty organization; on the board of Atkins Library; inducted in the UNC Alumni Hall of Fame, and on the Exponential Capital Campaign for UNC Charlotte. After my husband's death, with friends we endowed a scholarship for graduate nursing students and established an Interaction Lab with two-way mirrors so students can practice communication skills. Because of the support of my childhood sweetheart and husband of 40 years; best sister, Janice Sutphin; best friend, Laura Taylor; other friends, family, and colleagues I have been able to continue to contribute to my beloved university.

[Reflecting on being a faculty member] seemed so hard . . . it brought back a flood of both glorious and painful memories for me.

I loved teaching and I loved my students. As I see them at professional meetings as leaders, in the community as nursing leaders, and especially as colleagues who were once my students, seeing them do well still brings me great joy. As ANS advisor, I took students to the legislature; as UNC Charlotte faculty president, I helped usher in new gen-ed requirements; being awarded the Bank of America Teacher of Excellence early in my career gave me the opportunity to promote nursing educator as a wonderful career choice. My career came full-circle in developing and teaching an online program for preparing nurse educators and sending them out to teach nursing students across the state. However, over the span of a 34-year career, challenges were inevitable.

After over 40 years of being housed in the gym, scattered about on the campus (remember Denny 220), and 10 years in Colvard, we were ready to move into a beautiful new building as an interdisciplinary college. We had managed to land on our feet with the new structure. . . . We had swallowed the humiliation of being reduced to "school" status after we had been among the first five colleges at the university. We were ready to take nursing to a new level of influence at UNC Charlotte.

For most of us as faculty, teaching students to provide the best care possible was the #1 goal of our academic career. We are nurturing and caring by our nature, so fulfilling our service commitment to the university was something we excelled at as well. And we loved to share our posters and research findings with our nursing colleagues at local, state, and national meetings and conventions. A number of us even participated in "teaching circles" to share teaching exemplars. Although a number of faculty had small funded grants, getting big grants to fund research and writing scholarly papers in "tiered" journals had never been the basis for success in the College of Nursing. We were taking students to clinical, building programs on the backs of our master's-prepared faculty, providing service, maintaining a nursing clinic, and preparing students for the NCLEX.

After UNC Charlotte became a research institution in the early '90s, nursing's research program was still not well developed. Frequent changes in administrators (five deans plus two interims before we restructured, and two since) may have contributed. All of these things take a lot of energy even with a well-developed focused research program. And we were never able to find a CON/SON focus for research . . . so we were not keeping pace with the rest of the university related to its research mission.

Unfortunately we were not prepared for our first non-nursing dean. She was extremely well qualified, a researcher with prolific publications, seemingly everything we needed to jump-start our fledgling research efforts. But nursing never met her expectations. We had never before been led to believe that bringing in a certain level of grant money was the biggest factor in determining resources for the SON. I now realize how naive we were; we needed to cover our salary with grant money or lose resources for our department. We did not deal with it well and the dean did not either. I think neither of us realized how badly we needed nurturing in the importance of research and funding to secure nursing's future at the university. Hindsight can be painful.

We grew as a faculty during this period and produced an amazing group of students well prepared to care for patients in many settings. I am most proud of the number of nurse leaders who are 49er nurses. Research has become a part of their practice. Grants and publications have increased. Interim Director Dena Evans has employed an editor to assist faculty with manuscripts. Dr. Jackie Dienemann has described the remarkable research efforts of the faculty from our beginning in 1965–2017 in another part of this book.

I believe that the dreams of Miss Bonnie, Miss Edith Brocker, and Miss Elinor Caddell will take nursing to a new level of influence at UNC Charlotte. I'm betting on it!

SALLY REID GARRETT, CLASS OF 1970[14]

As I thought about writing this memory of my time at UNC Charlotte, many memories came to mind, but I decided to write about three of them.

When I began my nursing education at UNC Charlotte in 1966 there were no dormitories on campus. Those of us who were not "local" lived in the dorm at what was then known as Charlotte Memorial Hospital. In the beginning we shared the dorm with two other schools of nursing: the last class for the three-year diploma program at Charlotte Memorial, and students from the two-year Central Piedmont Community College program. So we had students from three types of schools of nursing living together. We often compared notes on our experiences and in the evenings we sat in the hallway, on the floor, and chatted and sang songs: one big happy family.

My second memory and one that I have cherished throughout my career was that of learning critical thinking from Ms. Elinor Caddell. Ms. Caddell had many wonderful qualities as an instructor but certainly the one that had the biggest impact on me was her ability to teach the art and science of critical thinking. Her exams were not just true/false or multiple choice but included scenarios that required the student to assess and think about what were the relevant facts and how did those facts impact your actions as a nurse. This skill has served me well and later in my career I was able to provide similar critical thinking training for nursing staff as well as develop competency measures to measure critical thinking. What a gift Ms. Caddell gave us.

The third memory I would like to share involves how our school pin came to be. The class of 1970 was the third nursing "class," but the previous classes were very small. Our class was small too, but at approximately 20 it was almost double the size of the previous class. The College of Nursing was so young that many of the traditions of a College of Nursing had not been established. We did not have a school pin. My roommate, Lynn Brown Dobson, and I sat in our room over several days drawing designs for a pin. Lynn, being the better artist, did most of the drawing. The design we came up with, with few changes, became the pin for the UNC Charlotte College of Nursing.

Most of my nursing career has been in inpatient psychiatric/mental health nursing, in public facilities with primarily indigent patients. I have held most every nursing position in a hospital, from staff nurse, manager, educator, to administrator. I ended my full-time career as the chief nurse executive at Northern Virginia Mental Health Institute. After retiring from that position I have been a nurse consultant, consulting with hospitals throughout the eastern United States. As my career winds down, I can look back and see the impact my education had, and I have a great appreciation for my UNC Charlotte College of Nursing experience.

LANNY ELLIS, MED, CLASS OF 1970[15]

I came to Charlotte after serving in the U.S. Navy as a hospital corpsman, along with my wife (an RN) and infant son. The Vietnam War was winding down at this time. My goal was to use the good medical training I received from the navy and enter nursing school at UNC Charlotte to obtain my BSN. The BSN degree was an important goal because (1) my wife had a BSN and (2) a BSN degree was a stepping-stone toward further advancement such as anesthesia, management, teaching, etc.

I entertained the idea of possibly going into anesthesia postgraduation from nursing school. One of my professors was Mrs. Vera Smith. Her husband was Mr. Eugene Smith, who was director of Nursing at Charlotte Memorial Hospital (now Carolinas HealthCare System) where we did our clinicals. Both had a very positive influence on me and my career. I later earned a MEd degree from UNC Charlotte.

I am extremely grateful toward my classmates for their acceptance and the support given me (a male "nurse") during the pursuit of obtaining my degree. We were a small but tight netted and supportive group, determined to reach our shared goals.

I retired from nursing in January 2014 after having practiced for 44 years. A challenging and fulfilling career in which I was able to practice my profession in a variety of areas: ER, major trauma, ICU, CCU, kidney transplantation, nursing supervision, and endoscopy.

All of this was made possible by the foundation set forth by UNC Charlotte School of Nursing, fantastic professors (Mrs. Edith Brocker, Mrs. Vera Smith, and Miss Elinor Caddell), and a wonderful group of classmates.

MARILYN G. SMITH, RN, MSN, CERTIFIED FNP, CLASS OF 1971[16]

In thinking about my student days at UNC Charlotte, it seems like just a few years ago, instead of 47 years ago that I walked on the campus as a transfer student. I went to a small religious university my first two years for a very sound reason. I was promised a car if I would go there instead of where I wanted to go, UNC Chapel Hill. I knew there was a university in Charlotte but didn't know anything about it. The boy I was seriously dating decided to go to Charlotte instead of Chapel Hill, so in the advanced wisdom of a then 19 year old, I started checking out the school and found out that they had a nursing program, and within a few months, I had given up my place at Chapel Hill, left a good friend scrambling at the last minute looking for a new roommate, and transferred to Charlotte in June 1969.

I had to go to summer school to catch up on a few of their requirements since some of their prerequisites were different than Chapel Hill's. After being at the university for about a month, my boyfriend, just turned fiancé, and I were driving to my home in Shelby. When we pulled up to my house, there were people and cars everywhere and one of my uncles quickly came out to the car and told me that my father had died in a boating accident. Everything after that was hazy. I think I went on automatic pilot and somehow finished that summer and started fall classes. Within a few months my fiancé and I drifted apart and the haze worsened. I'm not sure when the haze lifted, but I think it took much longer than a year. As I learned about grieving in the nursing curriculum, I realized that I was dealing with two significant losses at once.

I was talking to Elinor Caddell not too long ago and she said that she still remembered when my father died. I was shocked by that and told her how I didn't think I was going to make it. It was what she said next that to me epitomizes UNC Charlotte. She said that they (the faculty) were not going to let that happen! I graduated in a class of 12 students and remember very little about those two years, except how much I loved nursing, especially clinical care.

I got engaged again very quickly and married a month after graduation. I had been accepted to the master's program at Chapel Hill and decided to postpone that for a year while my husband finished coursework to transfer. I had decided to go to graduate school because of my admiration of Elinor Caddell. My thinking was that if graduate school could give me what she had, then that was what I would do. Little did I know that it wasn't graduate school that would make me like Elinor. I soon realized that she is truly an original!

I did go to Chapel Hill the following year and completed my master's in nursing in May 1974, two months after my son was born. After a short stint in Charleston, South Carolina, I moved back to Charlotte and a year later was contacted by Elinor Caddell about a teaching position. I had never planned on teaching, but because it was Elinor who called, I joined the faculty in 1977 and stayed until I retired in July 2008. During my years teaching at UNC Charlotte, I was able to complete the Family Nurse Practitioner program at USC Columbia.

I fondly remember other faculty including Edith Brocker, Joyce Lowder, Vera Smith, and Judy Mauldin. They all were so important to me and the other students and all had so much influence on all of our careers.

So, what did UNC Charlotte mean to me? Absolutely everything related to my nursing career I can give credit to Elinor Caddell and the other faculty. It is so rare to find the level of excellence and the intense caring I received during those years as a student, and later as a faculty member. My one desire when I started teaching was to give back some of what I had received.

LYNN DOBSON, CLASS OF 1970[17]

Prepared by Dona Haney

The following is reproduced from an interview with Lynn after she had won the 2015 UNC Charlotte Humanitarian Award. She was responding to the questions, "Describe your experiences at UNC Charlotte. What has this university meant to you?"

I was in the third graduating class. I had gone to the small Methodist school down the road, Pfeiffer, for two years and at the time they had a 2/3 program with Emory when I was ready to complete my last years, UNC Charlotte seemed a better place, closer to home; I am from a rural area 40 miles north of Charlotte and certainly less expensive. We had a small class and we all lived in the old nursing dorms attached to Carolina Medical Center. We really had more of a college life than most of the other students had as there were no dorms at that time.

The faculty was superb and I would say multitasked, to say the least. My most memorable faculty members were Joyce Lowder and Elinor Caddell. They taught us, mentored us as nurses and leaders, and they showed love and compassion. You see getting a BSN at that time was a bit new and at times all the students felt like they were being scrutinized for being academic and not practical enough. Ms. Lowder and Ms. Caddell taught us to stand tall in our knowledge and led by example. My senior year, I was president of our local student nurses' association and got a paid trip to the national convention in Detroit, Michigan. Most memorable because I felt I was prepared to communicate on the national level and even though at the time baccalaureate nursing degrees were outnumbered by hospital-based degrees, I could stand tall in my knowledge with the best in a variety of discussions.

The following information is also noted in the description of Lynn as the recipient of the Humanitarian Award.

- She received a master's of education from UNC Charlotte (1975) and served as a clinical instructor for UNC Charlotte from 1973–91. During that time she was one of three faculty members who started the nursing clinic at the Salvation Army for Women and Children.
- She then transitioned to a career of supporting women and children with cancer, including hospice, therapeutic childcare programs, mission work, and camps for special children.

- Emily Chiles who submitted her nomination for this award stated, "Lynn has an infectious, outgoing personality and entertains all who are around her. She is a very giving person, who reaches out to others, and especially those with physical needs and disabilities."
- She is a three-time cancer survivor.

Lynn was presented the School of Nursing Alumni Distinguished Alumni Award in 2015.

Lynn says, "My greatest accomplishment is marrying Bob Dobson and having Scott Dobson, a pediatrician in Greenville, South Carolina, with three grands, and Melanie Dobson, an ordained Methodist pastor with a doctorate in theology and youngest grand in Charlotte, North Carolina."

LUCILLE MOSES BSN, CLASS OF 1970[18]
Prepared by Dona Haney in consultation with John Moses

Lucille Moses was the youngest of 10 children; this included eight girls, five of whom would become nurses. Lucille graduated from Cumberland Maryland Hospital School of Nursing in 1943 and joined the Navy Nurse Corp.

Serving in the Navy Nurse Corp provided some special opportunities. She initially served at the Key West Naval Base where she took private flying lessons and achieved her goal of flying solo. She loved the view of the Keys from the air. One day, during an inspection of the barracks, the inspecting officer said, "Are you the nurse who flies the Piper Cub?" [When] she responded that she was, a fellow nurse asked her, "Why did he ask you if you flew a Paper Cup?" Due to some allergies she was transferred from Florida to Bethesda Naval Hospital. During this time, she took a course in Arabic at Georgetown University. Her interest in Arabic was related to both of her parents being Lebanese immigrants who spoke only Arabic. While at Bethesda, she met her future husband who was from a family of nine children and whose parents were from Lebanon.

In 1952 she left the navy to marry Dr. John Moses and moved to Charlotte. She raised her two children, but continued to pursue her love of learning, taking classes at CPCC, and, like many, hoped there would soon be a BSN program for the RN. It was her desire to teach nursing and having a BSN was required to fulfill this goal.

Upon learning that the program had become a reality, she promptly pursued admission. She had to take 30 credits hours at UNC Charlotte and take two nursing classes, Community Health and Nursing Leadership. Being an RN, in clinical she wore a white uniform and cap, unlike her classmates who wore the green student uniform. Lynn Dobson, a classmate, remembers her as "the elder statesman in the class." She graduated in 1970 in the third graduating class of the UNC Charlotte School of Nursing and became the first RN to receive her BSN from UNC Charlotte.

With her prior nursing experience, and the new BSN, she was now eligible to teach in the clinical setting. As Elinor Caddell says, "we were always looking for good candidates to teach clinicals." She was asked to become a part of the clinical staff. She developed the first laboratory of films and resources to support clinical education for the nursing students.

Consistent with her love of learning she obtained her master's in guidance and counseling and opened a counseling practice in Charlotte, which she maintained until her retirement.

Lucille is 97 years old and suffers from complications of aging. The information for this article was provided by her husband, Dr. John Moses.

KATHY WEBB (BARBER), CLASS OF 1970[19]

I have always been grateful to have chosen UNC Charlotte School of Nursing as my place to earn a nursing BS degree. The school had a small-school feel, yet had a large university standing. There were only 3–4 buildings on the UNC Charlotte campus when we started classes: Library, Science, Student Union, and Administration. I, along with a few other UNC Charlotte nursing students, including my twin sister–roommate, lived in the Charlotte Memorial Hospital School of Nursing dorm and saw the last class of the three-year nursing program graduate.

Our class had a strong educational foundation. The integrity and caring nature of the nursing instructors—Mrs. Edith Brocker, Ms. Elinor Caddell, and Mrs. Vera Smith—supported us throughout our training. Getting our uniforms in our sophomore year was a proud moment and the public nursing experiences were ones I have never forgotten. It was a part of the real world during our student training.

There was much change in the world scene and in education during the 1966–70 class years. By graduation, in 1970, UNC Charlotte was building a co-ed dormitory and other buildings on campus. Now it is a city on the outskirts of Charlotte.

As a final note, I met my husband through one of the nursing students. Her husband's best friend became my future husband. We were engaged right before graduation.

JANICE ELLIS, CLASS OF 1970[20]

During my years at nursing school, there was a feeling of unrest in the country. My future husband was in the army during most of my time in nursing school, and we got married a few months after I graduated. Intensive studies in the nursing program and concerns for my future husband were a constant theme during my years at the UNC Charlotte School of Nursing.

I loved the beautiful campus of UNC Charlotte—so new with only a few buildings and no dorms. We were housed at the dorm located next to Charlotte Memorial Hospital, which was quite convenient for student-nursing training. I roomed with my twin sister (also a nursing student). Our instructors made sure not to put us on the same floor or in the same rotation.

Mrs. Edith Brocker, Mrs. Vera Smith, and Miss Elinor Caddell were vibrant instructors who believed in giving their students a well-informed start in their nursing career. Our class, though small, was determined to finish strong and stand alongside the already established schools of nursing (UNC Charlotte, ECU, and Duke). Edith Brocker introduced public health nursing and pushed hard for accreditation for the new BSN at UNC Charlotte. Vera Smith and Elinor Caddell made sure we knew the nursing techniques and learned to think and assess patient situations. I could see the field of nursing was changing as new technology and computers were becoming a part of daily work life. After passing boards, I was happy to work in med-surg nursing and in a hospital-based clinic during my nursing career.

SUE HEAD, CLASS OF 1970[21]

I started at UNC Charlotte to acquire a BSN in 1969. I had previously attended Duke University School of Nursing for 3½ years. While at Duke I took a Nursing History class taught by Edith Brocker. Little did I know that I would later encounter her as the first dean of the School of Nursing at UNC Charlotte. In 1957 my family (a husband and a new baby) then moved to Texas as my husband had just completed seminary and had been accepted in postgraduate studies in Houston. It was common practice in that era for women to move with the family rather than the family moving while the woman finished her degree and my dear husband often stated, "My wife will never work."

In the late '60s, we returned to Charlotte. I now had four daughters and a husband very supportive of my finishing school to become a registered nurse. My husband had a professional association with Eugene Smith who was the director of Nursing at Charlotte Memorial Hospital. He told us of new programs at Central Piedmont Community College and at UNC Charlotte. I attended CPCC, completing their entire program to get my RN. I then met with Vera Smith (Eugene's wife who on the UNC Charlotte faculty) to discuss how to obtain a BSN. I entered the program and completed 30 hours of classes, as my original nursing courses transferred as collegiate credits. The two nursing courses at UNC Charlotte were Community Health and Leadership courses. I enjoyed going back to school as an adult; as an adult learner I found education both challenging and enjoyable.

Soon after graduation, I was called to a meeting with Mrs. Brocker, Vera Smith, and Elinor Caddell where I was asked to join the faculty as a part-time clinical instructor. During this three-year tenure (1971–74) I entered the master of education program at UNC. Not being satisfied with my educational attainment, I applied and was accepted to the graduate program at UNC Chapel Hill School of Nursing.

In 1974 I moved to Chapel Hill (weekdays only, my husband and daughters were still in Charlotte) to complete a MSN, which I completed in 1976, I then returned to Charlotte to continue teaching at UNC Charlotte. This was considered a bold move for a woman at this time, many of my friends were amazed that I would do this especially leaving four teenaged daughters in the care of a working minister-husband.

In 1976, I returned to full-time teaching at UNC Charlotte. I continue to be most passionate about the RN-to-BSN Pathways program, which was developed by Vera Smith and myself. Our first class started in 1979. The idea was to support the working RN by providing an educational experience which was based on the working nurses schedule and working experience. It was expected that the nurse continuing to work. The outline of the program mirrored the graduate program at Chapel Hill, which I had recently experienced. The curriculum philosophy was based on Knowles Adult Learning Theory. Students went to class one day a week, learning contracts were created based on the individual needs of the student, and clinical work was completed in the home setting with preceptors. We wanted individuals to develop creativity and critical thinking as they worked as teammates. I loved what we did with this program. The students felt it was a life-changing experience because they were involved in the learning process. I was excited when I could see the change and they could see it themselves. Several of the projects that began as a fulfillment of the requirement of the course would later be developed as very successful business models. The Pathways program ran from 1979–92 and continues as the RN-to-BSN program.

Another highlight of my career was going to England with a group of students from UNC Charlotte. My fellow educators on the trip were Vera Smith and Sally Nicholson.

A very difficult experience was dealing with a specific dean who was very disruptive. I was proud that we had enough faculty to stand up for what we thought was right. When our group met, we always would meet where we could be seen. When a vote of confidence was called, 19 of the 26 faculty voted "No Confidence."

Although there were lots of conflict situations, which can be described, the final straw began when the dean stated she was not renewing the contracts for several outstanding faculty. Her decision was made without due process as the procedure required.

The biggest influence on my career was Elinor Caddell. She has a true interest in students and their success. She was extremely creative about teaching and learning and a true need for inquiry. I continue to discuss items with Elinor, and recently we spent over an hour discussing a concept I would share with the Sunday school class I teach.

I retired in 1993 with many fond memories and many close friends. I am very glad that UNC Charlotte was a big part of my life.

LAVERNE HICKS MEYERS, RN, BSN, RETIRED OCN, CLASS OF 1970[22]

When I was in high school and began planning for college, I knew I wanted to graduate from a BSN and RN program at the same time. I knew myself well enough to realize if I only went to one, I would not enter and finish the other. I wrote Charlotte Memorial Hospital in 1966 and asked about their three-year program (goodness only knows why I wrote them). They replied they were in their last nursing class and I might contact Central Piedmont Community College or the University of North Carolina at Charlotte. I applied only to UNC Charlotte, and to my surprise, was accepted. Thus began my 48-year sojourn in Charlotte, North Carolina. I have never regretted that decision.

When I graduated in 1970, I began my nursing career as a private duty nurse to a newborn girl whose mother had lung and colon cancer. Little did I know that I would retire as an oncology nurse in 2014. The widower father was instrumental in getting me a job in an internal medicine office where I worked in various positions for the next 44 years. The original physicians' office included four physicians at the time I began working and grew to 14+. Throughout the following years, current happenings caused offices to merge and big businesses to buy them out. I began in a private office, merged with another, was bought out by Presbyterian Hospital; after 30 years in that system, I joined another private office with 8–10 doctors joining us at four locations. The predominant MD died, and the office was sold to the next "big" corporation, Carolinas HealthCare.

I began as an office nurse, assisting one doctor. Before state and federal regulations, I learned to perform various duties such as radiology, spirometry, front office, heart monitors, stress tests, phlebotomy, nurse manager of a satellite office; in other words, "jack-of-all-trades." The physicians included internal medicine, cardiology, pulmonary, infectious disease, gastroenterology, and finally, oncology. That became my love. I felt I had finally come home. I became oncology certified and had to renew the certification every four years. After working in this field exclusively for 25 years, beginning in office chemotherapy infusion and later as a doctor's nurse, I retired for health reasons, as many of us at this age find we have to do. At the age of 70, I still would like to work one to two days a week, but haven't found that dream position yet!!!!

The medical field began as private businesses and were like a patient's family. As time passed, it became specialized to include all disciplines and even more business-like. One had to struggle to make sure the patient was the center of care and not money and numbers. That meant going against some of the managed care ideas. Some offices survived like we did, and others could not survive financially. Today, the various disciplines are "owned" by big corporations, but are not housed together under one roof. They have their own sites and communicate through charts online.

Some graduates worked in the hospital all their nursing career, but I loved the day-to-day interaction of the patients through the office. Hospital nurses took care of them in a crisis, but I saw them as they struggled to survive daily. Also I was honored to interact with their families to make sure they were cared for properly.

During this nursing journey, I met my soulmate and we have been married for 44.5 years. He was in the air force at the time we were first married and Viet Nam was an ongoing nightmare. Thankfully he did not have to go there. We have two sons and eight grandchildren; they all live in this area. At the moment, no one has expressed an interest in becoming a nurse, but I am ready to push the issue if given a chance. I feel I made the right choice many years ago and do not regret that decision.

CHAPTER THREE

Conflict

Dr. Louise Schlachter, Dean, 1977–1983

Ann Mabe Newman, RN, PhD

Louise Schlachter, RN, PhD, came to UNC Charlotte from Pace University where she was a well-respected scholar and leader. The School of Nursing under her leadership is described as a period during which school leadership sought "to revise and redefine the philosophy and objectives of the BSN program"[1] in response to the needs of students and the community.

Dr. Schlachter wrote, "The 1978–79 academic year can best be described by noting it was a year of continued growth and transition."[2] Indeed, it was. Faculty responsibilities were restructured to clarify lines of communication within the College of Nursing (CON). The CON was beginning to show growing pains associated with moving from being one large faculty to faculty groups organized around academic and clinical specialties of faculty members, such as pediatrics, obstetrics, management, community health, psychiatric, and medical-surgical nursing. The concept of "course coordinators" was put in place with one faculty member from each specialty taking on the role of coordinating curriculum and course work for their specialty.

The RN Pathways program was fully implemented and graduated 29 students in May 1979. This program was created in response to a request from graduates with diplomas and associate's degrees who wanted to further their educations by obtaining a BSN. Professor Sue Head, RN, MSN; Dr. Sally Nicholson, RN, PhD; Professor Vera Smith, RN, MSN; and Dr. Pauline Mayo, RN, PhD were early innovative thinkers in making this program the success it became. For example, a few years earlier, as a BSN student, I was told that no credit would be awarded for my diploma from an accredited school of nursing. While I was disappointed, I agreed to serve as a student advisor on the RN/ BSN Program Committee. This committee suggested changes to the curriculum committee, which included awarding academic credit for courses previously taken by the RN. This program has continued to grow over the past 40 years and has produced many expert clinicians and leaders of civic and professional organizations. These valuable RNs moved the discipline forward in ways we never imagined when the program was first conceived.

The Outreach Program in Nursing, funded by the Area Health Education Center (AHEC), entered its last year in 1979. Six of the 11 students graduated in May 1979 and the last five in 1980. The closing of the outreach program was necessary to encourage application to our newly emerging master of science in nursing program. The MSN program was a goal first mentioned early in our history (1965) by our founding dean Edith Brocker. The faculty worked diligently to prepare the proposal for consideration by the appropriate university committees.

In 1997, during Dean Schlachter's tenure, she identified Professor Lucille Moses, RN, MSN, who was already on the faculty of the CON, to work with faculty to develop audio-visual media for student use. This early innovation may seem minor to us today with our sophisticated computers, online courses, and mannequins. However, at the time, this organized use of slides and tapes evidenced growth in the use of technology. Professor Moses was named as the first in the CON to hold the position of audio-visual clinician in 1979.

The College of Nursing offered nursing courses for credit at clinical agencies through the Continuing Education Department at UNC Charlotte. The course Ecology of Man was offered at Gaston Memorial Hospital for more than 30 interested staff nurses who wanted to earn their BSN. In addition to classes during the day, all nursing courses were also offered in the evenings.

The 1978–79 annual report also mentioned the increasing involvement of students as representatives on college committees and in community service.[3] Activities included a blood pressure screening in the community and a Red Cross blood drive.

Students were delighted with a new "pinning ceremony" held on the evening before the university commencement. They wore white uniforms and caps, walked across the stage in UNC Charlotte's McKnight Auditorium, and received their official nursing pin. Students were thrilled to participate and to have their families and friends at the ceremony and reception.

Student life was not all books and patient care. In December 1979, the Nursing Student Association in conjunction with the College of Nursing faculty held a banquet and dance for nursing students. And in April 1980, the faculty and junior students gave a picnic for the graduating seniors on the football field behind the gym. After refreshments, a volleyball tournament was held, and the students beat

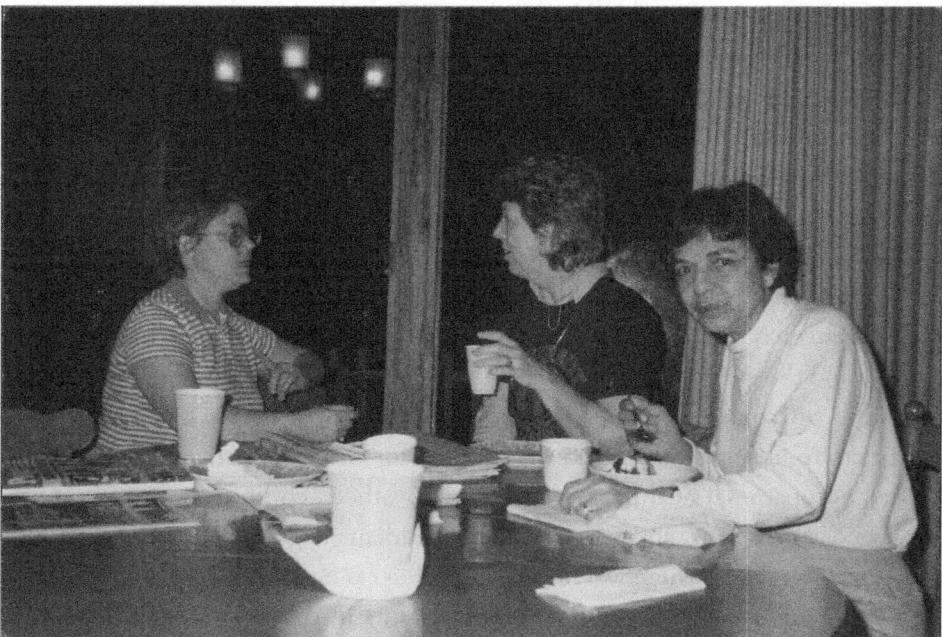

Lucille Moses with other faculty members Ann Newman and Frances King.

the faculty. Seniors received mean green ribbons and daisy corsages. One senior reported that it "was the nicest thing that anyone did during my time at UNCC."[4]

In the summary of her 1978–79 report, Dr. Schlachter noted that concerns about capitation funds and facilities loomed large. "The current state budget is woefully inadequate in view of the ongoing growth of the college," she wrote. "The College of Nursing is presently jammed into tiny makeshift offices in the gymnasium building. However, faculty are looking forward to moving into the new brick-of-the-month building, which is under construction, which will be available, hopefully, sometime during the next five years."[5]

Indeed, the College of Nursing was moved into spacious, new offices and classrooms in the Colvard Building in the summer of 1980. "The faculty and students are delighted with the well-planned, attractive facility that they are housed in," Dr. Schlachter wrote in her 1980 year-end report. During the Christmas holidays, the dean held a reception and tour of the Colvard Building.

Of more significance, however, was the implementation of the newly ratified criteria for appointment, tenure, and promotion within the College of Nursing. Until this time, faculty who were good teachers, shouldered their fair share of committee work, and participated in community service were usually tenured after their sixth year at the university. Many faculty members thought the process was administered arbitrarily, micro-managed by the dean, and did not reflect the philosophy of the faculty. While research and publication goals were important, the school was still in the phase of building programs, mostly on the backs of faculty with master's degrees who were not prepared to do research. Thus, several requests for faculty promotions and tenure were not forwarded to the next level. Several faculty resignations were accepted. This created a new source of tension between the faculty and administration.

Dr. Schlachter summarized the 1979–80 year by identifying the most serious challenges faced by the College of Nursing as "the paucity of state budgetary resources and the overuse of clinical facilities by many other health education units." In an effort to solve the problem of inadequate clinical space, the College of Nursing began to use sites other than the hospital for clinical practice. Other sites included occupational health offices, physician's offices, childcare centers, comprehensive day programs, and industrial sites. Students began to have opportunities to work with media, which was new to them. For example, videotapes of simulated home visits in which the faculty filmed students in role-play scenarios were recorded. The students then presented their tapes in class and their performances were critiqued.

A tradition was broken and a new one established in 1980. Until this time, students wore white uniforms and caps (RN/BSN students were allowed to wear the cap from their diploma or associate degree program) for the on-campus pinning ceremony held the evening before UNC Charlotte Convocation. "Nursing students will—for the first time—wear academic robes while participating in the Pinning Ceremony. Pins will be presented to students by elected faculty members. Fresh roses will be given to each graduate."[6]

"During the 1981–82 academic year the College of Nursing expanded and modified the programs in response to student and community needs," Dr. Schlachter reported in her annual review. The new undergraduate curriculum was reviewed and received accreditation for implementation from the NC State Board of Nursing. The Pathways program was recognized for its excellence by Governor James Hunt. The graduate program in nursing was approved for implementation in the fall of 1982. With graduate programs being offered, there was a renewed effort to recruit doctoral-level faculty.

Dr. Schlachter wrote in her 1981–82 annual report that "the College of Nursing faculty is developing into a professionally knowledgeable"[7] and active group. The 1981–82 annual report named outstanding faculty members who had received honors at the local, state, and national level: Professor Frances King, a delegate to the American Nurses' Association convention; Dr. Sally Nicholson, an advisor to

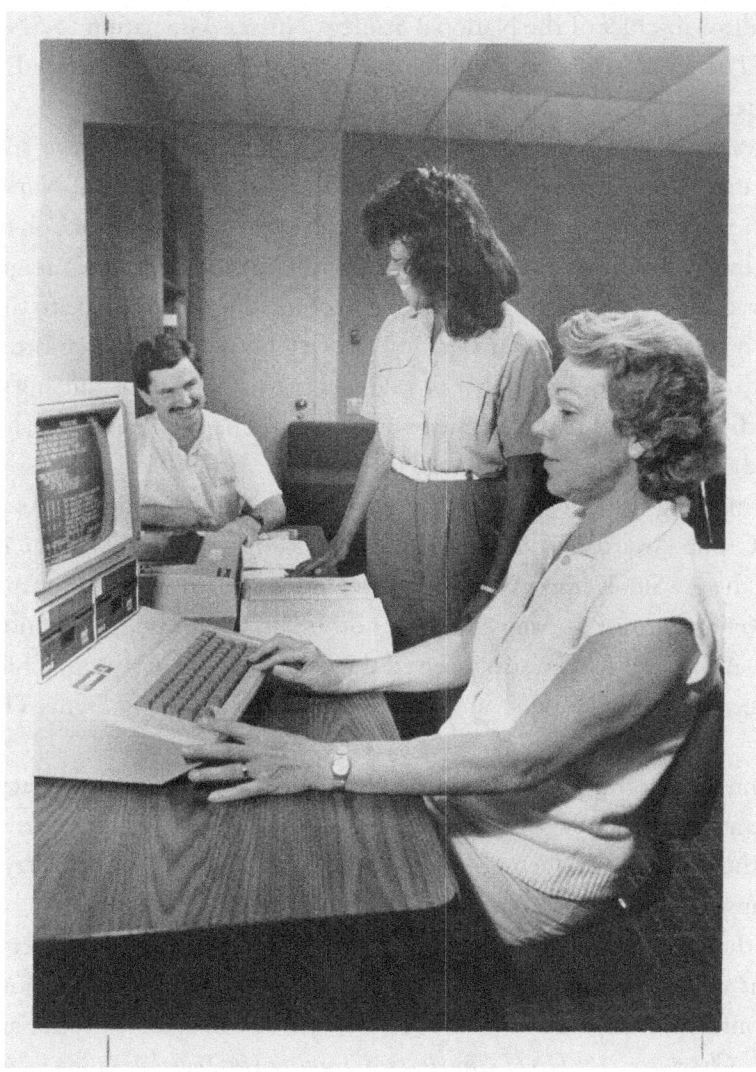

Nancy Hill with early graduate students.

the NC Association of Nursing Students; Professor Elinor Caddell, a member of the Health Services and who serves on its Board of Governors and was awarded the A. Sue Kerley Distinguished Professorship in Nursing; Professor Sue Head, a delegate to the Governor's Conference on Mental Health; and Professor Dorothy Schwobel, a delegate to the North Carolina Conference on Aging.[8]

Just as the faculty were growing and developing, so were the students. "Senior students organized and implemented blood pressure screenings on campus during Family Day, at Eastland Mall, at Tryon Shopping Center, and at Cotswold Shopping Center."[9] A UNC Charlotte College of Nursing senior, Sarah Brayboy, was named editor-in-chief of the National Student Nurses Association (NSNA) publication, *The Hypodermic,* and another senior was elected to the State Executive Committee in 1981.

The Seventh Annual Spring Luncheon and Lecture Series in 1982, co-sponsored by the Gamma Iota Chapter of Sigma Theta Tau and the College of Nursing, featured nationally known nursing author Dr. Beatrice Kalish, who spoke on the topic of "The Image of Nursing in the Mass Media." Students were encouraged to be "media watchers" and report negative images of nursing in the media to the ANA. Dr. Kalish and Dean Schlachter were interviewed by WBTV in Charlotte.

In May 1982, the largest number of students in the College of Nursing's history graduated—184—and 18% graduated with honors. The Auxiliary of the Mecklenburg Medical Society funded an award for Excellence in Nursing. The award went to senior nursing student Suzanne Miller, who also won the Alumni Association Interest Group Award. Senior nursing student Kathy Anderson, from Charlotte, received the A. Sue Kerley Award for Psychiatric Nursing. The dean-sponsored awards went to senior nursing students, both from Charlotte, Mary Gibson Lee and Rose Ann Leakan, who also received the Dean's Award in Parent/Child Nursing and Leadership in Nursing, and the Gamma Iota Chapter of Sigma Theta Tau Award.

In summarizing the year, Dr. Schlachter said, "With the support of faculty and administration, the College of Nursing has been able to meet its objectives as set forth in the April 8, 1981, memorandum to academic affairs."[10] The objectives were met because of the dedicated faculty.

Over the next couple of years, conflicts arose between Dr. Schlachter and the faculty, as well as university administration, which culminated in a majority vote of "no confidence" in the dean. The conflict was summarized by Ken Sanford in his book, *Charlotte and UNC Charlotte: Growing Up Together* (1996). "As in the economy, there were a few rough spots in the academic arena," he wrote. "After a period of some academic turmoil, Louise Schlachter left the deanship of nursing and returned to the classroom in 1983."[11]

Dr. Schlachter died in 2008 in Williamsburg, Virginia, at the age of 89.

CHAPTER FOUR

A Year of Healing

Dr. Pauline Mayo, Acting Dean, 1984–1985

My two years in the life of the College of Nursing. Did it make a difference? The record will show that many changes did occur during this brief time. Some of these changes included hiring more qualified faculty, finishing and implementing a new undergraduate curriculum, continuing a new graduate program, and consulting with nationally known educators. Consultants included Dr. Carolyn Waltz from the University of Maryland who helped develop a plan for systematic evaluation of the curriculum. Five new faculty with excellent academic credentials were recruited including Dr. Bea Chase, Dr. Mary Curran, and Dr. Kathleen Boggs, as well as two well qualified minority members, Bettie Gordon and Carol Fray.

From my perspective, these very positive changes were not the most important ones. The goal was to change the culture of the college to one of trust acceptance and freedom to pursue individual and shared goals. Also, this was a time in my life where I was focusing on physical fitness and emotional and spiritual growth. Therefore, I was concerned with the health of the faculty. We did some exercise and yoga as a group at noon on some days. These were fun and bonding activities. During this period, I was able to run a marathon, which was one of my personal goals.

The first graduates of the master's program in adult health graduated in August 1984. The RN Pathways degree program continued to attract large numbers of nurses from the area and an extension program was planned to be implemented in Gastonia during the 1985–86 academic year. The faculty commitment was obvious as they carried on with scholarly activities, participation in numerous workshops, alumni affairs, and professional and community activities. Faculty were also active in college and university committees, including the dean's search committee. Lienne Edwards, Sue Head, Marinell Jernigan, and Ruth Mauldin served on this committee chaired by Dr. John Lincourt of the Philosophy Department.

The more than 400 nursing students were also active on college and university committees and Sigma Theta Tau, while maintaining high levels of academic and clinical performance.

The focus for the spring of 1985 was on selecting and interviewing candidates for the deanship. I submitted my name at the urging of some faculty members, although I felt that my job was finished and the college was in excellent shape to move forward with new leadership. It had been an honor to serve as acting dean and to represent the college at community, state, and national meetings. Calm had been restored, trust and healing had occurred, and the college was ready to move forward. Yes, I believe that I made a positive difference!

Student Memories, 1980s

DEEANNA L. BURLESON, CLASS OF 1982[1]

At the age of five, I decided I would be a nurse. By that very early age, I had experienced three eye surgeries and experienced the care of a nurse. The care of a nurse meant someone I knew who was there to attend to any expected or unexpected need such as a stuffy nose. Although I did not like those nasal drops going down the back of my throat and I cried, I knew I was cared for as a child. Now, I tell people I was born a nurse and that is what it feels like even to this day. I do not ever remember not being a nurse and caring for people, animals, or the environment.

My experience and training at UNC Charlotte's School of Nursing was a critical part of what my future would hold, but first I would like to give a quick description of my journey to that point in my professional and personal life. For several reasons, when I was 16, I consciously decided I wanted to get married. At the age of 17, I gave birth to my first beautiful daughter and at age 20, my second beautiful daughter. Although not the most conducive way to achieving an education or a future career I would not change having my two daughters for an easier path to my dream career. During these early years of motherhood, I finished high school earlier than the planned path, trained to be a nursing assistant, and completed a Licensed Practical Nurse (LPN) program at Stanly Community College in Albemarle, North Carolina. I always knew I wanted to become a registered nurse and never lost sight of that dream.

My professional education continued at Stanly Community College in a joint, collaborative program with UNC Charlotte where I could take my basic college courses such as English, Biology, and Math. Finally, I could begin my nursing studies at the Charlotte campus and a whole new world opened. I was the type of student for which the university was created. Yes, it was a struggle; by this time, I was a single mother of two and working as a LPN in our local emergency department. I often started my evening studying after 9pm when my daughters were asleep. And yes, odds were, the night before a test, one or both would be sick, needing more attention than normal. I have to give a big shout out for my mother, Margaret Burleson, who helped so often in caring for my children when I needed assistance to meet all the requirements in my life. In addition to accomplishing my childhood dream, I was motivated by accomplishing something that would allow me to provide a better life for my daughters.

Through the experiences provided in my nursing program at UNC Charlotte, I saw many new possible doors in being a nurse. The options seemed to be endless in the areas of home care, intensive care, patient education, and even the military.

After I completed my bachelor of science in nursing (BSN), I continued to work as a registered nurse in the local emergency room. The nurses who had encouraged me, although I think there was always a thought of can she really do this being a single mother, continued to be there. The first time I started an IV on a patient, they were all at the door watching and probably holding their breath. I am very thankful for those nurses who were such a support to my success in completing this professional nursing program.

In addition to working in the emergency department, I joined the local Air National Guard and trained to be a flight nurse. To my surprise, the chief nurse of this unit was the assistant dean from the UNC Charlotte School of Nursing, Sally Nicholson. I could never have dreamed what my future held for me in the civilian and military sectors of health care.

My civilian nursing career included experience in several types or sizes of emergency departments, intensive care units, and homecare agencies. It included experiences as clinical nurse, administrator, risk manager, and program evaluator. My military career included experiences as a flight nurse on two types of aircraft and many types of deployments and training exercises. I held a top secret security clearance and conducted bio-surveillance activities interacting with all federal agencies that held bio-surveillance data. I retired as a Lt. Colonel after 26 years with my last assignment at the Pentagon with the Joint Staff Surgeon General as a staff assistant. Wow, who saw all those opportunities in 1982 when I completed my BSN?

My education continued, not just with the education I obtained in the facilities I worked and the military certifications, but I was able to achieve a masters in nursing with a focus on executive nursing from the Medical College of Virginia in Richmond, Virginia. I had experienced a disconnect between what we did to run our nursing units, what the patients and staff needed, and how to even ask for what we needed to provide the essential care, thus the reason I chose a program that combined nursing with healthcare administration.

In all my various types of work experiences I continued to see patients, families, and even staff suffering because of gaps and fragmentation in our healthcare systems. So, I decided to combine all my experiences and my passions and complete a PhD in organizational systems with a focus on patient-centered care and creating cultures of health and well-being for patients, families, and staff. Health care, those we care for, and those who provide care are all examples of complex systems creating one of the most complex systems in our society. These complex systems require complex solutions and that is where I am today as I write this summary of my career and the impact that the UNC Charlotte School of Nursing played in my career and professional life. Now I am involved with researching, coaching, team development, and sharing new ways of thinking about real health care. Doing whatever I can to help move our healthcare system to one that is truly about the health and well-being of the individuals involved.

SUSAN HUDSON MARSTON, CLASS OF 1982[2]

1982 was the year of *An Officer and a Gentleman,* Michael Jackson's *Thriller* album, and the first Jarvik artificial heart implant. I did my nursing clinicals at Charlotte Memorial Hospital, Mercy, and Gaston Memorial Hospital. I remember during my pediatric rotation at Charlotte Memorial, I met a wonderful peds resident and was so impressed with how he interacted with the children. Luckily he stayed in Charlotte and that resident, Dr. Tim Eichenbrenner, became my children's pediatrician. I remember my psych rotation at Gaston and the first time I had to care for a colostomy patient at Charlotte Memorial. I had studied all night about how to care for the patient and perform colostomy care. I wasn't prepared for it and the smell really affected me to the point that I had to excuse myself and almost fainted in the hall as I slid down the wall with my instructor. I remember the Kardex system they had at Mercy at that time.

Unfortunately I failed chemistry and had to repeat it during the summer. One day I stopped by the candy store on campus and got some jawbreakers. I dropped some during class and I remember the professor saying how he hated teaching chemistry in the summer because we were all nursing students that had failed and not chemistry majors. One of my favorite classes by far was anatomy and physiology. One of the best places to hang out was the Belk Tower. I was so saddened when I visited there recently to learn it was taken down due to deteriorating conditions. It was such an iconic structure to me. The campus in the early '80s was so small and quaint. I loved the student lounge and the game room where the PacMan, Tetris, and DigDug video games were always in use. I was a commuter and we had to park in one of the only lots there and now the space is huge with parking decks. The growth is phenomenal.

On a sad note, I remember a dear classmate of ours was tragically killed on I-85 going home from work after the night shift. The day she was killed was the day we received our letters in the mail and she never knew she had passed her boards and was officially a nurse. I still remember how impressed I was by her natural nursing skills. Back then we had to wait for our notification in the mail and depending on the size and shape of the letter you knew if you had passed or failed before you even opened the mail.

The UNC Charlotte School of Nursing prepared me for the wonderful career I have had. I have been with Carolinas HealthCare System for 35 years and have truly enjoyed every minute. I have gone back to get an MBA and worked in various areas including med-surg, ortho, pain management, endoscopy, OR, and the physician practices in positions from staff nurse to nurse manger to director of various areas. UNC Charlotte taught me all the skills I needed to have a successful and long nursing career and I am so thankful I had to opportunity to attend. I am still in contact with some of those classmates who are still with CHS.

NELLA LINKER, CLASS OF 1989[3]

I was a RN-to-BSN student. My 46 years of nursing, when I retired, were in public health; eight of those years were in correctional nursing.

The BSN program at UNC Charlotte allowed me to remain in public health. Because management and public health required a BSN, I was able to enhance my career with the BSN degree I earned at UNC Charlotte.

UNC Charlotte taught me an entirely different perspective to public health and made me a better nurse. Thank you UNC Charlotte School of Nursing.

ROBYN HILL TURTON, CLASS OF 1982[4]

Nursing was a second profession for me having been a social worker for several years. When I decided to go into nursing, a co-worker's husband who was a CRNA recommended I go to UNC Charlotte rather than Central Piedmont as he said the BSN will soon be the entry degree into the profession. I took his good advice and found UNC Charlotte not only an academically challenging environment, but also a place where I made lasting relationships.

In a class of 100 students, I became acquainted with three other older students and we stayed remarkably connected throughout nursing school. Two of us remained in Charlotte after graduation and the other two had nursing careers in Raleigh and Georgetown, South Carolina. My friend who lived and worked in Charlotte and I started our nursing careers together, attended conferences and graduate school together, and remained close friends until she sadly passed away in 2005. I keep her obituary in my wallet still today. My friendships with other 1982 UNC Charlotte graduates grew as we started our careers at Charlotte Memorial Hospital (now Carolinas Medical Center). Susan Hudson Marston and Cindy Brenton, both 1982 graduates with whom I've worked, have accomplished much in their long and respected careers.

The faculty at UNC Charlotte encouraged professional growth, community service, and high standards. As a former Sigma Theta Tau, Gamma Iota chapter president, I was one of the original organizers of the Mecklenburg County Organization of Nurses annual banquet to celebrate nursing still held every May and supported by the local hospitals, specialty clinics, and professional nursing associations.

Over the years I kept up with Ann Newman, PhD, who facilitated my psych/mental health field placement. She taught us about being "change agents," and the importance of nursing leadership in the community by her community service, letters to the editor, and running for state AORN and Board of Nursing offices. UNC Charlotte faculty also managed community clinics for the underserved.

I am grateful to have had a long and rewarding career in nursing and could not have chosen a better launchpad than UNC Charlotte!

LYNDA COLVARD OPDYKE, CLASS OF 1984[5]

I had been a nursing educator for more than 20 years with a full-time job. I was a wife and mother and active in the community.

There was pressure from nursing education accrediting and approval agencies that all faculty must hold at least a master's degree.

Because of political issues, the UNC system was slow to approve expansion of MSN programs in North Carolina. My family and job responsibilities prevented me from commuting to Greensboro or Chapel Hill for graduate study. I joined an effort to contact the consolidated university officials and emphasize the need for graduate nursing education in Charlotte. I was almost finished with graduate work in education when the MSN program was finally approved. I switched majors and became a member of the first MSN class at UNC Charlotte.

Thanks to UNC Charlotte, I was able to complete a successful career in nursing education. While enrolled at UNC Charlotte, I became interested in healthcare ethics. I was a charter member of Mercy Hospital's ethics committee, did postgraduate study in healthcare ethics, and chaired the city's Bioethics Resource Group. At this time, the College of Nursing was housed in the newly completed Colvard Building.

DATRA DELK-PATRICK, CLASS OF 1987[6]

I am excited to be part of UNC Charlotte's nursing history!

My goal in life was to become a nurse, just like my Aunt Janie, who was a nurse. My aunt advised me to choose a BSN program (wonderful advice!!) and to look at the NCLEX pass rates of the schools I was considering. I remember that UNC Charlotte had a very high pass rate, and that made an impression on me. I applied and was accepted and entered UNC Charlotte as a freshman nursing major. At that time, we were able to declare our major as a freshman. The first years were filled with getting the general education courses, learning how to live away from home, making new friends, and getting excited about starting the nursing courses. I can remember the day that I went to the bookstore to buy my first nursing textbooks. I was so excited to buy all of those big books!! We used the buddy system when we went to the bookstore to buy books and help each other get them back to our dorm (Sycamore Hall). Once we got into the flow of the classroom content and passed our skills labs, we were ready to take on the hospital!!

Our clinical group would pack in the car and head down I-77 to Charlotte Memorial Hospital to get our clinical assignment the evening before clinical, and then back to UNC Charlotte to work on drug cards, care plans, and trying to learn as much as possible so we could survive the next day at clinical! One of my favorite clinical days was my OR rotation. I was able to observe an abdominal case and then follow the patient to recovery (PACU). I learned from that experience why patients experienced pain other than at the incision site, such as pain from the use of retractors and devices to enable better visualization of the operative area, and the importance of proper positioning on the OR table. Clinical was hard, but what and how I was taught made the biggest impression on me. I remember a particular day in clinical that I was struggling with some things and Ruth Mauldin, my clinical instructor, pulled me into the supply closet. I thought I was finished, but she looked at me and with her kind sternness told me that she knew I could do this, that I had great potential, and that I needed confidence in myself. That helped tremendously and helped me get through the clinical day and gave me the confidence I needed to pass the NCLEX the first time I took the exam.

I have a very fond memory of one day in our Psych-Mental Health class, we were all feeling like we could not do nursing any more, and Dr. Ann Newman came in for our lecture. She put down her books/notes and looked out over our class and said, "I know this is hard, I know you all are working hard, and I can see that you are looking stressed. I just want you to know that I believe in you and that you can get through this and be good nurses." After her pep talk, she invited us all up to get a "warm fuzzy." She had a blue ceramic jar with the inscription "Warm Fuzzies" and inside were yellow cotton balls. I carried my warm fuzzy in my notebook for a long time and anytime I felt stressed, I pulled out my warm fuzzy and reflected on what Dr. Newman had told us. I also have fond memories of OB content with Dr. Lienne Edwards, Community Health with Ruth Stephenson, Informatics with Dr. Curran, and Public Health with Dr. Guttman.

In addition to our nursing studies, we were encouraged to be part of the Association of Nursing Students (ANS). Our advisor was Dr. Ann Newman and she always told us how important it was to be part of our professional organization and to always keep learning and growing. Dr. Newman was a member of the North Carolina Nurses Association (NCNA) and would share information with us from her meetings. I was honored to be the president of our ANS chapter my senior year. At our last ANS meeting of the year, the ANS members and faculty presented me with a plaque with the inscription, "In appreciation for demonstrating those qualities of leadership and friendship that give us excellence today for a better tomorrow." That plaque hangs in my study and is a constant reminder of the wonderful experience I had at UNC Charlotte. That experience in ANS has proven to be very valuable as I have been a member of the North Carolina Nurses Association for 30 years and held several different offices at the local level. It is also pretty cool that I still get to see Dr. Newman at the state NCNA conventions!

During my time at UNC Charlotte, there was a very sad time that touched all of us, that was January 28, 1986, when the space shuttle Challenger exploded after takeoff. I remember that cold January day and there was a quiet over the campus for the days to follow. I'm sure we talked about it in class the following day, but we were mostly just in disbelief that it happened.

UNC Charlotte School of Nursing has had a great impact on my nursing career. After I graduated and passed my boards, I started in Women's Services, and after about two years on 12-hour nights, I needed to see daylight so I took a position in public health for a few years. After my OR experience in school, I still had the desire to work in the OR, so I took a position back at the hospital in the OR and loved it. I was fortunate to move up the ranks and took the position of nurse clinician for Women's Services and Surgical Services. After I completed my master's in nursing education, I accepted the position of clinical nurse educator for the hospital. I spent 15 years in clinical education but wanted to try education from the academic point of view. I was offered and accepted a nursing faculty position at our local community college teaching in the associate degree program. This has been the most rewarding position that I have had in nursing! Currently, I am an assistant professor of nursing at Davidson County Community College, where I am the lead instructor in the LPN-to-ADN Transition option, which is taught online and I have clinical students who are precepted across the state. I am also the lead faculty for our nursing program accreditation. I can definitely say my education at UNC Charlotte provided the foundation and experience that has helped me grow in my nursing career.

TERESA D. PARKER, CLASS OF 1984[7]

What was going on in the world or in the community that had an impact on you, your education or your career? There were lots of firsts—first test tube baby, Sally Ride became the first American woman in space, Sandra Day O'Connor was nominated as first female justice on Supreme Court, and the AIDS virus was discovered.

UNC Charlotte professors had a huge impact on making me the nurse I am today and I owe them much thanks—Ann Newman, Marilyn Smith, Glenna Davenport-Cook, Emily Chiles, Lienne Edwards; they made me strive to be the best that I could be in the classroom as well as in clinical. I remember going to class all day on Tuesday and Thursday, leaving campus and driving downtown to Charlotte Memorial Hospital (now CMC Main) to get my assignment for the following day, going home, and researching the diagnoses of the patient as well as all the medications the patient was taking, do a care plan on my patient, and being prepared to answer questions first thing the following morning for clinicals on Wednesday and Friday.

The quote I remember from then is: "A mental health day is as important as any physical sick day you will ever take."

Some of the other things that were happening during my time at UNC Charlotte were: JR was shot on Dallas, Luke and Laura got married on General Hospital, Princess Diana and Charles got married, and Cabbage Patch dolls and PAC-Man arcade game were popular. Our student nurse uniforms consisted of a green dress with a white apron over it and we always wore our nursing caps which we were so very proud of!!! Charlotte only had ~300,000 people in the 1980s. I typed all of my college papers on a typewriter—never touched a computer! Highway 74 was known just as Independence Blvd and was simply a four-lane highway with multiple stoplights and shopping centers along the way. Had never heard of a cell phone.

I currently have my own business, RN4U, a senior advocacy and case management business—my strong UNC Charlotte nursing professors/leaders taught me that anything is possible in nursing and helped me to achieve this.

DELORES WONG, CLASS OF 1985[8]

I'm Delores Wong, graduate of the 1985 class of UNC Charlotte School of Nursing. My journey to UNC Charlotte was not a direct path from high school graduation in 1975 to UNC Charlotte. I attended UNC Greensboro for two years as a pre-nursing major, then transferred to Appalachian State University, where I graduated in 1979 with a BA in English. After moving to Charlotte in 1980, now married, but bouncing from one clerical position to another, I decided that I would finish my nursing prerequisites and go to nursing school.

I went to CPCC—Central Piedmont Community College—for one year to finish all of my electives and prerequisites for the nursing program at UNC Charlotte and transferred in as a junior in the fall of 1983.

Although trying to juggle part-time jobs and going to nursing school full time was difficult, I found that I loved being back in school and through some friends I had made at CPCC, plus some new-found friends after I transferred, I made it through. I remember the large classroom in the nursing building where we had our lecture classes, and I remember putting on the green dress uniform with the white pinafore and nursing cap and nervously going to clinical for the first time! Most of all, I remember so many wonderful, supportive, and encouraging faculty members—and a few that struck fear into our hearts (they shall remain nameless)! A few names of faculty that I remember—Ann Newman, Marinell Jernigan, Lienne Edwards, and of course, Elinor Caddell! Lynn Dobson had us rolling with laughter as we practiced our physical assessments on each other! Marilyn Smith was my favorite med-surg clinical supervisor, and she was always so encouraging and instilled confidence in us that we could take care of our assigned patients. I looked online to see how many, if any, faculty that I knew, are still working for UNC Charlotte. There are not many, but I did see that we have some male nursing faculty now! We didn't have any of those in 1983–85, although we had probably about 5–10 male nursing students.

I graduated in 1985, with a plan to work in the Dickson Heart Unit at Charlotte Memorial Hospital, now Carolinas Medical Center, however a job opportunity for my husband changed all of that. He took a new position that required us to move to Elkin, North Carolina, which was my hometown, and my first nursing position was at Forsyth Memorial Hospital, now Novant, in Winston-Salem. I remember that back then, until we passed boards, we worked as "graduate nurses," making what now would be barely above minimum wage.

Since that time, I have worked at Iredell Memorial Hospital in Statesville, North Carolina, for Kaiser-Permanente in Charlotte (yes, I did end up back in the Charlotte area—moving to Gastonia, North Carolina, in 1991 with my husband and two children), and for the past 17 years, I've worked with many other UNC Charlotte alumni, for Gaston Memorial Hospital, and now with CaroMont Health in Gastonia.

Wherever I have been employed, I have always been proud to wear my UNC Charlotte nursing pin on my badge and to state that I'm a graduate of UNC Charlotte. Thanks to all of my nursing professors, both classroom and clinical, who instilled in me a love of taking care of people and the ability to see the whole person.

CONNIE MELE, MSN, RN, PMHCNS-BC, CARN-AP, NE-BC, FIAAN, CLASS OF 1984[9]

I was living in Cleveland, Ohio, and my husband and I decided to relocate to the South. I always knew I wanted to return to school to get my BSN, so I started looking for nursing schools that had 2+2 programs. There were five. I visited all of them and decided UNC Charlotte's program was the one I wanted to go to. So we moved to Charlotte in 1979 and I began taking classes in 1980. I had to take a number of classes before I could get into the 2+2 program. And as most students in the program, I was working full time. At this time, I was working in addictions nursing. I felt very fortunate to have found my "niche" in nursing. What I appreciated about the Pathways program was I got to do all my clinical work in addictions nursing. It was also during this program that I began to understand the importance of being involved in my nursing organizations such as the North Carolina Nurses Association. It was at this time I was given the opportunity to serve on a new committee that was being formed on dysfunctional families. I felt drawn to this committee because it was an opportunity to become an active member of NCNA and to use my knowledge and expertise. In essence it allowed me to give back to my profession. From this committee the NCNA Peer Assistance Program was formed to assist nurses with substance use disorders. It was exciting to be on the ground floor of the development of this program. I would not have had the confidence to "put myself out there," if it had not been for my coursework and the encouragement from my professors in the Pathways program.

After I finished my BSN, I took some time off before deciding to return for my master's degree in psychiatric/mental health nursing (class of '95). I decided to return in 1990. At the time, I thought I would like to go into private practice to help people. I had been working in treatment facilities for addictions for 11 years and thought I would enjoy working with people "one on one." As I went through my program, managed care began to become more prominent in behavioral health services. I wasn't sure that I wanted to spend my days doing paperwork vs. helping people. I also realized that nursing students were not getting any education on how to treat the patient who had substance use disorders. And yet, any place that they went to work, they would encounter people with alcohol and drug problems. So I decided to focus my thesis on developing a nursing class that not only would give them the knowledge they need to effectively treat them but it also evaluated their attitudes about people who had the disease of addiction. As we all know, stigma is one of the downsides to seeking treatment for it. I continue to teach this class each semester to the nursing students at UNC Charlotte.

In addition, I continued to do work on behalf of nurses with substance use disorders. I got involved in my specialty organization (The International Nurses Society on Addictions) at a board level. It was through my coursework and my faculty advisor, Dr. Ann Newman, that I felt compelled to do more than just be a member of the organization. She instilled in us that we truly "needed to be the change that we wanted to see in the world." Whether it was advocating for those who could not speak for themselves or encouraging nurses to become involved politically—whatever it was—we could not nor should not sit idly by. It has become the philosophy upon which I have built my nursing career.

In addition, the school gave me one of my greatest treasures. My best friend Kathy Partney (class of '84) Shields. We were in an elective course on grief together, she was a post-op nurse and I was a nurse working in chemical dependency at the time. We would have never met if it hadn't been for that course. She and I became fast friends. She was from Pennsylvania and I was from Ohio. While our paths in nursing weren't the same, we were so much alike in other ways. We even celebrated our graduation together by having one party. We were like two peas in a pod. Kathy and I are still best friends today, even though she got married and moved back to Pennsylvania. (What was she thinking?!?!) We get together every other year with our husbands for a long weekend visit in a new city and state. What fun we have!!

CHAPTER FIVE

Regrouping, Moving Forward, Hitting Our Stride

Dr. Nancy F. Langston, Dean,
College of Nursing, 1985–1992

It was my privilege to join the faculty of this young university and College of Nursing in 1985. During my first year, a major focus became continuation of the work started by the interim dean to heal the internal chaos that had developed in the college. In order to address the chaos and breach of trust between the faculty and administration, I communicated with the faculty directly and often, and encouraged everyone to "say what you mean, and mean what you say."

In addition to this significant work on communication and trust-building, the faculty and administration began to focus on the school's mission. To that end, we boldly stated in our strategic plan that we would make ourselves an indispensable unit of the university by assuring congruence between our work and the unfolding development of this young university. During the first 20 years since Miss Bonnie established this urban university, the primary focus had been on the development of its portfolio of academic programs and degrees. Scholarship, research, and community service were only beginning to emerge as part of the vision.

During my relatively short tenure at the college—six years—I found the faculty eager to engage in significant new ways of thinking and being. We, as a faculty, actively embraced the emerging tripartite mission of the university. We engaged in enhancing the quality of our academic programs and expanding their impact and influence, and developed new skill sets within our faculty to assume this expanded vision of our work.

In regard to our academic programs, we continued to offer robust programs at the undergraduate and graduate levels. During the late 1980s, there was a

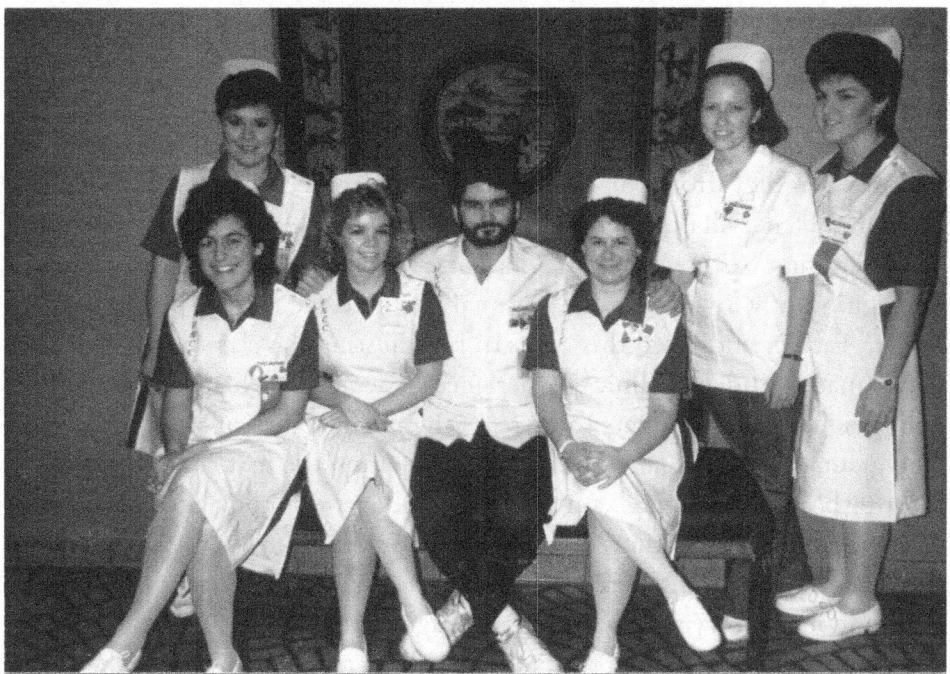

Students at 1988 NC Association of Nursing Students Convention in Greensboro.

focus on increasing enrollment in the undergraduate program's generic and pathways tracks. Additionally, in the generic track there was a focus on student success, as measured by licensure pass rates. Simultaneously, we began a comprehensive curriculum review with the goal of implementing a new upper-division nursing concentration in the fall of 1991.

In 1985, the college was on the leading edge of increasing access to academic programs for nurses prepared in associate degree and diploma programs. The pathways track was truly innovative, and its course of study is now common among nursing programs throughout the nation. Our creation of a seamless process for furthering the education of these nurses and building upon their basic programs rather than duplicating much of their basic content and clinical experiences was an exemplar. During my tenure, the primary focus for the Pathways program was to disseminate information about this "new program" to educational programs throughout the region and to expand outreach to prospective students.

For our undergraduate program, there was a two-pronged focus: increasing enrollment and enhancing program quality and student success. In 1988, faculty began a comprehensive curriculum review and revision with the goal of having a new upper-division major passed through all approval processes in time for the fall of 1991. Faculty also implemented instructional strategies to increase the first-time pass rate of new graduates on the licensure examination. Licensure examination pass rates for the UNC system became a political liability for the system when they dropped below the pass rates touted by community college programs. Hence all nursing programs were under intense review by university administration. Although UNC Charlotte's College of Nursing pass rate was not significantly lower than the national pass rate, we felt the pressure to "do better." Faculty addressed this concern by adjusting the classroom content to better match students' clinical experiences. Faculty also focused on working with graduates and students to increase their probability of success; students who graduated in 1988 and failed the examination the first time were offered tutoring before taking the exam again. All students who took advantage of this offer passed the second time. For the 1989–90 academic year, a specific within-curriculum plan was instituted to include standardized testing mid-year for seniors and mandatory review sessions throughout the last semester for students who scored below a set score on standardized test components. Over the course of three years the pass rate increased from the 1980s to the mid-1990s.

Another focus was on increasing enrollment in the face of impending major nursing shortages. Throughout my six-year tenure a variety of strategies was instituted, including extensive advertising in local newspapers and conducting open houses for students at UNC Charlotte who were undecided on their majors. These activities proved ineffective in increasing enrollment to the target levels established for the college. Thus, in 1989–90, we offered a part-time position for an individual to convert inquiries to enrolled students in the generic and the pathways tracks. This strategy, combined with the increased national focus on nursing as a high-demand career opportunity, resulted in a dramatic increase in enrollment; in the upper division, enrollment even exceeded projections for the 1990–91 academic year.

At the graduate level, our focus was on enrollment growth and program extension. Enrollment in the graduate specialties of the college was declining in the late 1980s. Faculty conducted focus sessions with enrolled students as well as other individuals who did not accept offers of enrollment in an effort to identify issues behind the declining enrollment. One major issue that emerged was that our program was not viewed as competitive with other programs in the state because our program required more credit hours than other programs. Faculty reviewed the curriculum for options to reduce credit hours and determined that several of the research courses could be eliminated from the curriculum, given

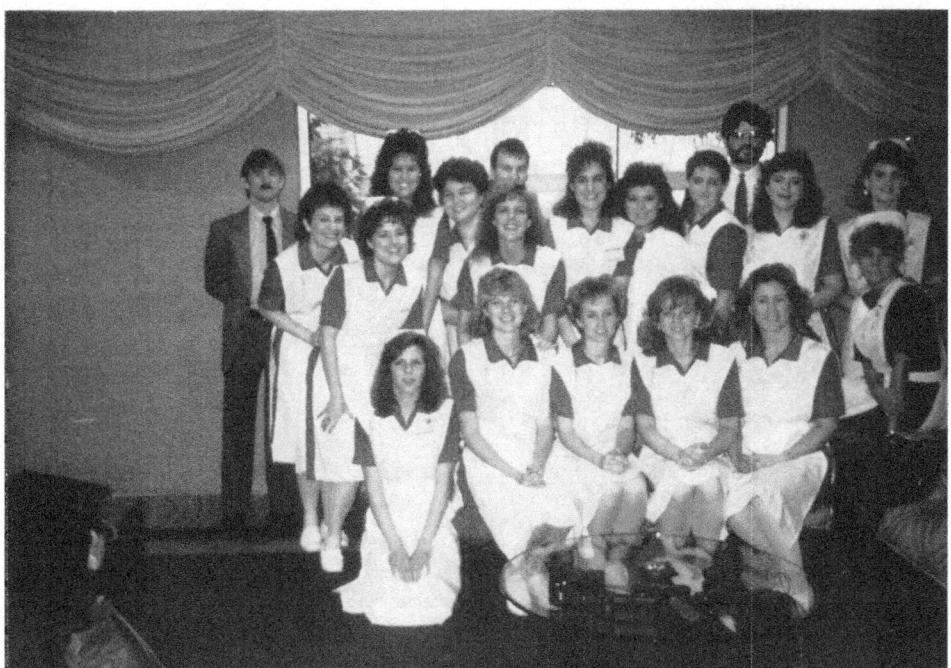

Students at State Convention.

that independent research was no longer an expectation for master's-prepared nurses. Hence in 1989–90 the graduate program credit hours were reduced from 45 to 38. In addition to this curriculum modification aimed at increasing enrollment, the college accepted a challenge from the NC Area Health Education Consortium program to provide graduate program access to baccalaureate-prepared nurses living in the far western part of the state. The college worked with the Asheville AHEC and the University of North Carolina Asheville to offer a hybrid program combining televised classes from Charlotte and onsite clinical experiences in Asheville. The adult-health/teaching concentration was selected as the course of study for this outreach program. The only new faculty appointed was a part-time nursing position to supervise the clinical practicum in Asheville. Additionally, the nursing director of the Asheville AHEC sat in on every course and class as it was televised in order to ensure that transmission and reception was smooth and effective. In 1988–89, 28 students enrolled in this outreach program.

In addition to these revisions and innovations, faculty worked with the hospital-based nurse anesthesia program housed at Carolina's Medical Center to move the CMC program into the graduate nursing program at UNC Char-

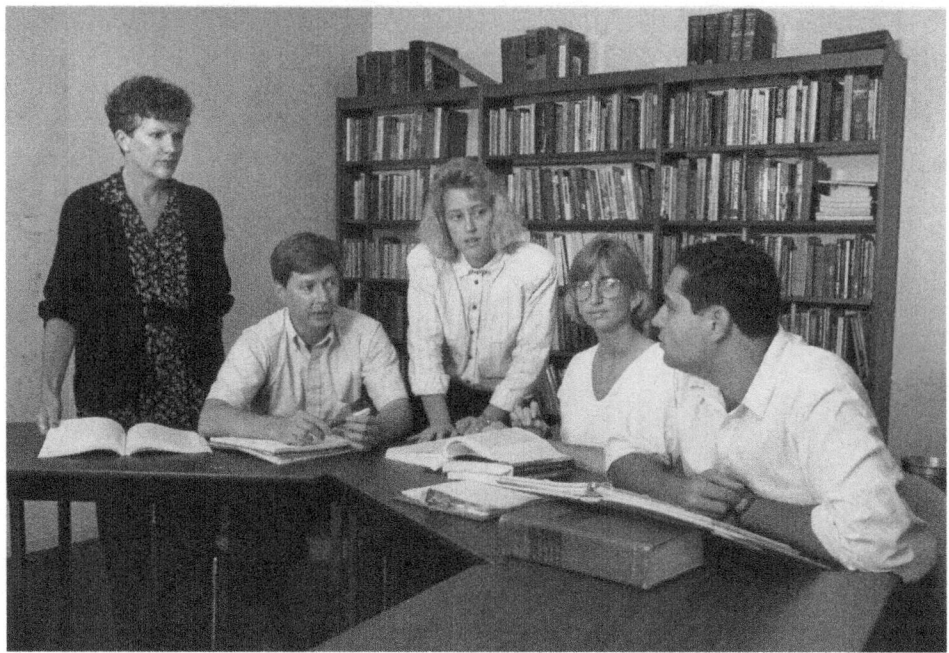

Anesthesia students.

lotte. Again, the college was on the cutting edge of work to move nurse anesthesia education into the mainstream of higher education while maintaining the integrity, strengths, and cultures of both programs. The melding of cultures across institutions and student groups was challenging and time-intensive; hence a coordinator from the college was appointed to guide this work. The first cohort of 12 students was admitted in the fall of 1988 and graduated in 1991, achieving a 100% pass rate on the CRNA licensure examination.

The faculty had a long-standing history of engaging in the traditional service work of the academy of nursing by serving on numerous committees and task forces. During the late 1980s, faculty began to expand the definition of service to embrace the idea of using one's professional knowledge to serve the profession of nursing as well as to provide clinical services in new ways and to traditionally underserved populations. Based on their volunteer work at the homeless men's shelter clinic, two faculty members who were nurse practitioners identified an unmet need in the community. Based on their observations, they noted that very few homeless women sought care at the clinic at the men's shelter. They undertook a project to understand where and how homeless women accessed care. As a result of information gained during this assessment, they developed a part-time on-site clinic at the shelter for homeless women. As the clinic matured, it also served as a site for select experiences for both undergraduate and graduate nursing students. In addition to providing direct clinical services, faculty began to serve on the boards of health-related organizations in the community, such as a hospice organization, the local March of Dimes, and the NC State Health Coordinating Council. This clinical work and community service advanced our profession, raised our profile in the community, and improved the health care of our neighbors.

Prior to the mid-1980s, the primary focus of the university had been on instructional programs and institutional infrastructure development. However, when I became dean, university-level discussions had begun regarding the need for research as the "third leg" of the university's tripartite foundation. Thus, we began the conversation within the college about what our discipline's scholarship should be and our faculty's commitment to it. These conversations led us to conclude that faculty should begin work to publish manuscripts derived from reflective analysis of their current activities in clinical practice and professional service. In short order, our focus shifted to include the importance of conducting research to generate new knowledge. This expansion in thinking about scholarly work led to the appointment of a faculty member with a joint appointment to a local hospital in order to stimulate clinically relevant research projects and to build a bridge between the college faculty and clinical agencies. Additionally, a faculty member from UNC Chapel Hill School of Nursing who was nationally renowned as a writer and editor was retained as a consultant to assist individual faculty in development of manuscripts for publication. This awakening focus combined with the beginning of systems of support for scholarship and research resulted in a large increase in the number of faculty involved in publishing and the number of publications/presentations produced in 1985–86 and 1990–91. In 1989–90, there were seven refereed presentations, and in 1990–91, there were nine refereed presentations and five more scheduled for presentation. In 1989–90, there was one refereed article, and in 1990–91, there were six in print and two accepted for publication. We had been successful in embracing a new element of our mission.

I have long held the belief that unlike businesses that adhere to the tenet, "no margin, no mission," the appropriate slogan for a university is "no faculty, no mission." Hence a significant focus during my time as dean was to support the faculty. Excellent teachers or clinicians, who had no desire to advance beyond their current master's degrees, were supported in that work. Faculty who wished to obtain advanced degrees were supported in those endeavors, and new faculty with doctoral degrees were recruited. The composition of the faculty in terms

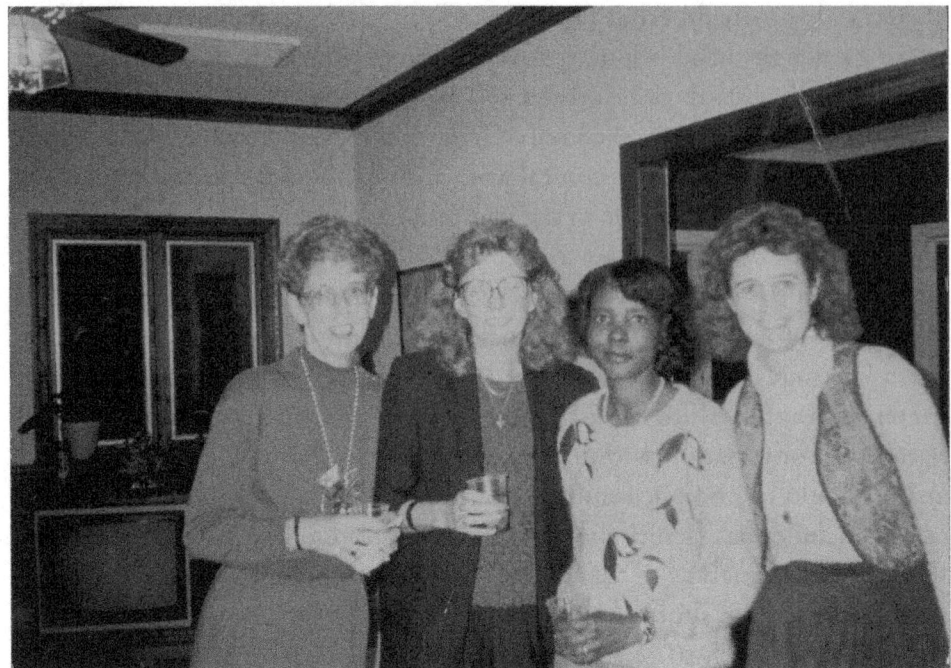

Four faculty celebrate their new PhDs.

of academic preparation changed dramatically from 1985 to 1991. In 1985–86, there were 32 full-time faculty members including the dean. Of those, 10 held doctoral degrees, two of those were in nursing. In 1990–91, the full-time faculty was still 32; however, 23 now had doctoral degrees, 10 of which were in nursing.

As I reflect upon my six years at the college, I am in awe of what we accomplished together. It was a pleasure to work with faculty who were so passionate about their work as educators and willing to step out on the leading edge of innovation to make both undergraduate and graduate programs accessible and of high quality. It was a privilege to work with faculty members who were willing to envision new ways of being together in their work and, in fact, envision new work for themselves and their colleagues. I left after six short years, not because I wanted to leave UNC Charlotte, but rather because I was drawn to the challenges of a nursing program that provided a full range of academic programs, from BS through PhD, and that was located in an academic health sciences center. I believe I was far more successful there than I would have been had I not had the privilege of working with the great faculty at UNC Charlotte SON in an environment that was young, vibrant, and willing to embrace a new way of being and working. I am grateful for the time we had together.

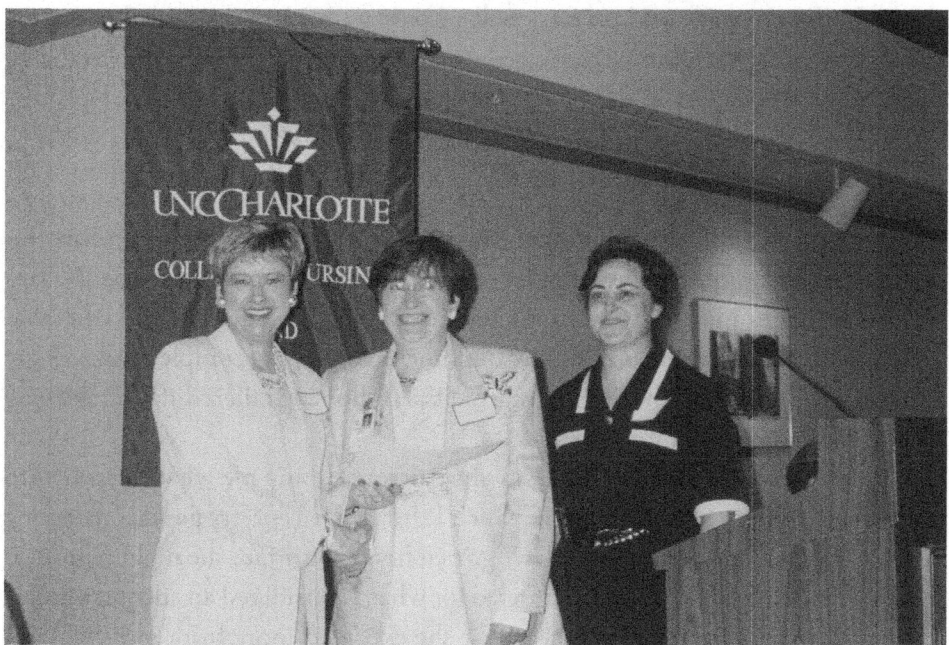

Spring Lecture, Dona Haney, Pat Campbell, and Trish Heatherly.

Student Memories, 1990s

EILEEN A. CURRAN, CLASS OF 1998[1]

- Received RN at CPCC.
- Transferred to UNC Charlotte to complete BSN.
- Was a nontraditional student (40 years old) with two children and a husband (who travels).
- Commuted one day a week for classes all day and additional day of clinical
- This was a very tough time in my life trying to hold everything together.
- Other than class time, I did not spend any other time at UNC Charlotte.
- There seemed to be plenty of opportunities to socialize and join clubs and associations, I just didn't have time for any of that.
- I did find the faculty very professional and supportive (and flexible).
- Unlike my time at the community college, many students were older with family and work responsibilities in addition to college.

Personally, as I look back, I don't know how I did it. Luckily, I had a very supportive husband. But, I am very glad I did it. Having my BSN has helped me in many

ways—both personally and professionally. I only wish I had continued to get my
NP. There is a tremendous need for geriatric NPs and I would have enjoyed being
a part of that need.

CHRISTIAN CARBALLO, CLASS OF 1998[2]

UNC Charlotte, and much of Charlotte's university area, was still a growing institution when I stumbled into it in December 1994. I remember eating at the Ap-
plebee's within minutes of the campus, looking at the then-unfamiliar red dirt that
surrounded the restaurant as they were building the shopping complex and wishing
I were someplace else. When school started that following fall, it did not take long
for the school to change my mind.

I remember Tama Morris, one of my instructors, asking me what happened to
my grade in our first exam. I had a B, which I thought was pretty good considering
I didn't really study and I may not have gotten home until 3am the night before, so
I was surprised that I was being counseled for what I considered an adequate grade.
She was very kind but also very clear that she expected more from me—which I
produced, at least for the next exam before bad study habits and the general dis-
tractions of college life won over.

It is this delicate balance of growth and caring that I found to be unique and
truly special. The school was certainly growing; we had to enter the library from
the back because a new entrance was being built, and the Fretwell building would
soon be constructed, but although campus expansion and increasing the student
population was an obvious goal, the faculty acted like it was a small school. Rather
than navigating my way through a maze of secretaries and TAs, you knocked on a
door and just talked to the people teaching the class—that is if they don't catch
you in the hallways first. There was certainly a sense that the faculty believed that
students were people rather than faceless occupiers of seats in the classrooms, which
was probably why we had Dr. Moore showing up to our final Pharmacology exam
wearing a witch's hat that was half as tall as she was, alleviating some of the stress as
we marched into the final exam of what was the hardest class that semester.

The school I never wanted to attend won me over. Enough for me to come back
for another bachelor's degree and a graduate degree, all great experiences and all
very instrumental in establishing a basis for me, not just as a professional, but as a
father and a man.

CHAPTER SIX

Managing Change in 1992–2004

Strategic Planning, Assessing, Restructuring, Building, Merging, and Moving

Dr. Ina Sue Marquis Bishop, PhD, RN, FAAN

In the fall of 1992, the College of Nursing began a season of dramatic changes that continued for more than a decade. The scope of change was broad and deep. It encompassed organizational structure; faculty governance; academic programs; technological advances; revisions in strategic planning and evaluation; expectations and roles for faculty, staff, and administrators; community outreach; and changes in the physical environment. These changes were in concert with ambitious changes in the university under the leadership of Chancellor James Woodward and the recently appointed Vice Chancellor and Provost Philip Dubois. Forces at work in nursing education and in healthcare delivery systems also had implications that would result in major changes in UNC Charlotte's School of Nursing.

Energy was high during these years as faculty and administrators revised long-range strategic goals, projected areas of growth and change, and planned actions to achieve goals. While these changes were readily embraced, they were also a source of stress and uncertainty. Leadership during this period of high growth was focused on managing change—planning, effective communication, involvement of faculty and staff, implementation, and evaluation. Listening, creativity, and a sense of humor were orders of the day.

The goal in the first years of restructuring was to bring leadership and accountability to needed areas. In many cases, resources weren't available for full-time positions or full implementation of plans. In subsequent years, as budgets allowed, full-time equivalents (FTE) could be allocated to specific positions. Meanwhile, much could be accomplished in two to four hours a week. So, value was added in increments as everyone worked toward long-range goals.

Throughout the 1990s and beyond, strategic plans were updated every five years and evaluated on an annual basis. This process was utilized fully to spur continued growth and excellence in the college and to make a successful case for additional resources from the university and external sources. There is little doubt that the strategic planning process initiated by Woodard and Dubois was the engine fueled by effective communication and creative collaboration. These were exciting and busy years.

An Evolving Organizational Structure

Sue Marquis Bishop, RN, PhD, assumed the position of dean of the College of Nursing on July 1, 1992, when the majority of faculty were on nine-month appointments and away on summer recess. On the new dean's desk was an action voted on by the faculty prior to leaving for the summer—to create academic departments in the college.

The proposed restructuring was congruent with the university's organizational structure of colleges with academic departments that brought together scholars and teachers in shared specialties. Many other colleges of nursing were undergoing similar restructuring. Multiple nursing specialties lent themselves to this kind of organization that could potentially create benefits for teaching and research.

Certainly, there was some risk in establishing three new academic departments only a year before the graduate and undergraduate nursing programs would be reviewed for accreditation by the National League for Nursing (NLN). The NC State Board of Nursing also planned to visit the baccalaureate program in the coming year for accreditation.

While interest was high for departmentalizing and there was compelling rationale for doing so, when Dean Bishop arrived, there was only the vote to go ahead. There were no open positions available for department chairs, and the necessary revisions in bylaws and faculty governance to support the reorganization had not been developed.

In the first month after she assumed her position, Bishop consulted with each faculty member on the proposed reorganization, soliciting recommendations for department leadership positions. It was clear that the reorganization needed to be implemented this year or postposed for two years until the NLN reaccreditation visit had been completed. The consensus was that the potential benefits in moving forward with departmentalizing outweighed other considerations.

Creating academic departments in the College of Nursing was a significant undertaking, especially in such a short time span. It required moving faculty physically into new spaces, writing new position descriptions, revising faculty governance, developing evaluation procedures, and creating committees—all at the same time that the accreditation self-study and the North Carolina Board of Nursing review were in process—and with new administrators at every level.

Provost Dubois supported the plan to create academic departments in the College of Nursing and allocated three new positions in support of the proposed reorganization. When faculty returned in August 1992, a draft of the new organizational structure was available, plans were underway to recruit nationally for department chairs, and a timeline for actions to implement the decentralization of the College of Nursing was ready for faculty review. In August, prior to the start of classes, faculty retreated to a cabin in Uwharrie Forest to set goals and make plans for the coming year. They met in academic departments for the first time and continued to meet monthly during the year.

The 1992–93 academic year began with the goal of fully implementing the reorganization. The graduate coordinator position was upgraded to associate dean for Academic Affairs, and Barbara Carper, RN, PhD, was appointed. Dr. Carper had served with distinction as interim dean in 1991–92 during the national search for a new dean. She assumed administrative responsibilities for the student services area, working closely with the new Office of Student Services (OSS), the Nursing Skills Learning Center, and the nursing curriculum committees. Pamala Larsen, RN, PhD, was appointed as associate dean for Academic Affairs in 1999.

The reorganization established three academic departments to be chaired by three interim department chairs: Department of Adult Health Nursing (Marinell Jernigan, RN, EdD), Department of Parent Child and Women's Health Nursing (Lienne Edwards, RN, PhD), and the Department of Community Health, Psychiatric Mental Health and Nursing Systems (Janice Janken, RN, PhD. By the fall of 1993, two department chairs had been recruited. In the Department of Community Health, Psychiatric Mental Health Nursing and Nursing Systems, Sara Torres, PhD, RN, FAAN, was appointed chair. In the Department of Parent Child and Women's Health Nursing, Irma D'Antonio, PhD, RN, was appointed chair and served for three years until she retired. Debra Hymovich, RN, PhD, served as interim chair for a year following Dr. D'Antonio's retirement. Dr. Jernigan continued to serve as chair of the Department of Adult Health Nursing until her retirement in 1997. She was replaced by Leslie Hussey, RN, PhD.

During the 1992–93 academic year, collegial efforts to establish effective and ongoing communication were critical in enabling faculty, administrators, and staff to successfully meet strategic goals and manage significant changes. The new administrative team—dean, associate dean, department chairs, directors, chair of the

Faculty Organization, and administrative assistant—met weekly in the fall semester and monthly in the spring to facilitate communication. Staff development was made available to help administration team members with their roles in the new organization. The staff was solicited for suggestions to improve the effectiveness of college operations. And, information about upcoming activities was disseminated. An ad hoc steering committee led preparations for the NLN self-study report for MSN and BSN and BSN Pathways programs (RN/BSN).

By the spring of 1993, the College of Nursing's Mission Statement was revised and long-range strategic goals were developed. In retrospect, it was truly amazing how much was accomplished in these early watershed years.

Historically, in the College of Nursing, administration of financial resources was centralized in the dean's office. In support of the new de-centralized organization, departmental budgets were established for department chairs to administer, and to the associate dean for Academic Affairs for the Office of Student Services and Nursing Skills Lab.

In 1997, the decision was made that nursing programs and research would be better served as part of the Department of Parent Child and Women's Health Nursing with the Department of Community Health, Psychiatric Mental Health Nursing and Nursing Systems. In the fall of 1997, Bill Cody, RN, PhD, was appointed chair of the newly integrated department, renamed the Department of Family and Community Nursing. In the initial phases of reorganization, unit titles were long, as no one wanted their specialty to be left out; over time, as faculty worked together, department names were shortened.

Strategic Planning

As strategic planning at the university progressed in the 1990s, there were occasional discussions about moving academic units from one college to another. Chancellor Woodward initiated such a discussion in a meeting with Dean Bishop when she was a candidate for the position. He indicated he would welcome ideas on how to organize healthcare disciplines to maximize the development of education and research programs.

Faculty recognized the potential benefits of collaboration in teaching and research in a multidisciplinary health college. However, there were serious concerns about restructuring the school into a multidisciplinary college: (1) Nursing programs had always been located in the College of Nursing. What would it mean to lose the identity of an independent academic unit? Would this be a hindrance in recruiting new faculty? (2) The creation of a multidisciplinary college had implications for future appointments of deans, who might not have nursing backgrounds. (3) State and national accreditation guidelines stipulate that the dean of the College of Nursing is responsible for administering nursing programs. How would this be addressed in the future?

Dean Bishop met with the dean of the College of Education, who recommended moving the Department of Health Promotion and Kinesiology (HPK) to a multidisciplinary health college. Dean Bishop also met with the chair and faculty of HPK. Faculty were also amenable to the move. They saw commonalities in health professions education and clinical practice, as well as opportunities for multidisciplinary teaching and research, but were concerned about promotion and tenure reviews. The College of Nursing and HPK faculties met to name the new college and settled on the "College of Nursing and Health Professions (CNHP)."

On July 1, 1996, HPK faculty moved from the College of Education to the new CNHP. HPK kept their physical location in the Belk Gym since their labs were located there. The mission and vision statements and faculty governance systems were revised to fit the new multidisciplinary CNHP.

The University Health Commission

A new vice chancellor and provost, Denise Trauth, PhD, was appointed to replace Provost Dubois when he resigned to take the position of president of the University of Wyoming. Provost Trauth had previously served as dean of the Graduate School. In 2000, a University Health Commission was appointed to provide leadership for long-range strategic planning. Commission members represented the College of Nursing and Health Professions, College of Arts and Sciences, and Belk College of Business. Dean Bishop was appointed co-chair along with Dean Bob Mundt, PhD, dean of the Graduate School, and Distinguished Professor of Health Policy, Bill Brandon, PhD. All faculty were engaged in extensive discussions.

College of Nursing faculty agreed that: (1) If the College of Nursing were restructured within a multidisciplinary college, it was critical that the nursing programs be organized in a School of Nursing and retain the current two academic departments: Adult Health Nursing and Family and Community Nursing. (2) The administrative head of the School of Nursing should be appointed to associate dean and director of the School of Nursing. This recommendation would address any concerns from accrediting bodies.

During the year, the commission reviewed available data on program needs in the state and region, considered strengths and resources at UNC Charlotte, interviewed key leaders in community healthcare settings, and presented mini-position papers for discussion. The co-chairs traveled to the University of Central Florida and the University of Connecticut to meet with faculty in multidisciplinary health colleges and departments to discuss issues and challenges.

After a year of evaluation and strategic planning, a final Health Commission Report was submitted to Provost Phil Dubois and formally presented to the University Faculty Council. The report included long-range goals for proposed academic programs and a recommendation to further expand the multidisciplinary College of Nursing and Health Professions to a College of Health and Human Services. On March 22, 2002, the UNC Charlotte Board of Trustees approved the College of Health and Human Services (CHHS). Later that same year, Pamala Larsen, RN, PhD, was appointed as the first associate dean and director of the School of Nursing. Jane Neese, RN, PhD, was appointed associate dean of Academic Affairs.

Laying the Groundwork

Academic units in the new college initially included: School of Nursing (with the departments of Adult Health Nursing and Family and Community Nursing), Department of Kinesiology, (formerly in the College of Education), and the Department of Social Work (moved from the College of Arts and Sciences). A new Department of Health Behavior and Administration (HBA) was created. Management of the multidisciplinary master's program in Health Administration (MHA) was moved from the College of Arts and Sciences to the new HBA department, but faculty from three colleges would contribute to this multidisciplinary graduate program. Andrew Harver, PhD, whose research focused on asthma prevention and treatment for children, moved from the Department of Psychology to serve as the first chair of the HBA. Subsequently, the master's program in Health Promotion was moved from the Department of Kinesiology (formerly Department of Health Promotion and Kinesiology) to the HBA.

In August 2002, the multidisciplinary health sciences and human services faculty convened for the first time. Once again there were new colleagues, new initiatives, and new challenges, but an atmosphere of energy and enthusiasm prevailed. Academic departments and committees reviewed and updated bylaws, faculty governance, and procedures for faculty promotion and tenure reviews. They wrote new mission and vision statements as well as five-year strategic plans. Plans were also being made as to how centralized services in the new college would support all academic units: Office of Student Services, Office of Research, Director of Continuing Education, Director of Health Informatics Lab. The College of Health and Human Services' new primary goal, mission, and vision statements are described below.

College of Health and Human Services Primary Goal[1]

The College of Health and Human Services (CHHS) aspires to excellence in educational programs, scholarship and research, and community service in human services and health sciences.

Vision Statement of the College of Health and Human Services[2]

The College of Health and Human Services promotes optimal health and high quality of health care and human services in the state and region through diversity and excellence in educational programs, research, and community service, including continuing education and clinical practice. The college recognizes the interdisciplinary nature of the health and human services professions and contributes its creative resources in partnership with individuals and institutions in the region to address the changing needs of healthcare and human services.

Mission Statement of the College of Health and Human Services[3]

The College of Health and Human Services offers professionally recognized and accessible undergraduate and graduate programs that are nationally and globally relevant, and responsive to changing needs of healthcare and human services in the state and region. The college achieves excellence through informed and effective teaching in its degree programs, continuing education, community outreach services and partnerships, professional activities, and research to advance science and practice in the health and human services professions.

Establishing an Office of Student Services

An assessment of college goals in 1992–93 indicated that specialized leadership and additional resources were needed in student services. In 1993, Dr. Bettie Glenn, RN, PhD, nursing faculty, was appointed director of Student Services at 30% FTE. Initially, she was charged with leading development of a centralized Office of Student Services (OSS) in the College of Nursing. Other positions were brought in to support OSS: the Academic Counselor position was upgraded from a 9-month to a 12-month position, and a Secretary III position was upgraded to a Records Clerk IV-59 and assigned 50% FTE to the OSS. All graduate, undergraduate, and pre-nursing student records were moved to the new centralized office. Student records were evaluated and updated, a new filing system devised, handouts for various programs created, new procedures and policies for student services implemented, and a computerized student data system devised.

In 1994, group advising for pre-nursing students was offered. A Student Evaluation of Advising Survey was developed by Academic Counselor Doug Hatcher, and students in six classes were surveyed (77% response rate). Students reported their faculty advisors were interested in them (72%), were helpful (97%), but only 25% reported their advisor seemed knowledgeable about policies and procedures. The OSS utilized data from the survey to plan workshops for faculty on policies and procedures.

In 1995, off-site recruitment and advising for BSN-RN and MSN students was offered in regional hospitals. OSS staff also had contact with 4,800 potential students at the NC Nurses Association, National Student Nurses Association, and the National College Fair.

In 1999, the OSS completed a survey of 500 undergraduate students in the college. Results indicated they were satisfied at the level of very good to excellent with the academic advising they were receiving. A survey of graduate students in 2000 and undergraduates in 2001 revealed students were highly satisfied with the assistance they were receiving from advisors. Further, a student database was devised to track individual students in all academic programs and to provide aggregate information on demographics for each program in the College of Nursing and Health Professions to assist academic departments in decision-making.

In 2000, a survey of employers from area medical centers was conducted at Gaston Memorial Hospital, Carolinas Medical Center, Presbyterian Hospital, and Northeast Medical Center regarding their satisfaction with BSN and MSN graduates. Clinical managers completing the survey indicated high satisfaction with UNC Charlotte nursing graduates (4.1 for BSN and 4.2 for MSN on a 5.0 scale). They indicated the strengths of graduates included: "knowledge, critical thinking ability, self-confidence and ability to prioritize." A suggested area for improvement for BSN students was "increased clinical experiences."

In 2002, new policies required by clinical institutions for student placement were implemented. They required drug testing for social work, nursing, and athletic training students, and criminal background checks.

During 2003, a three-year follow-up survey was conducted of baccalaureate program graduates, indicating that 22.5% of 2000 graduates were enrolled in graduate programs.

The OSS continued to develop over the years to become a major resource for the college. In the 1990s, the office was singled out by on-site visitors from various accrediting bodies for excellence in providing services to prospective and current students, support for faculty advisors, program outreach, advising, and data collection to evaluate effectiveness.

Improving Instruction in the Nursing Skills Learning Lab

The Nursing Skills Learning Laboratory (NSLL) is a vital learning lab for the nursing programs, used primarily by the BSN program in 1992. In 1992, Delores Sanders, RN, PhD, was appointed as the first coordinator of the Nursing Skills Learning Laboratory. Goals for the first year were to assess and enhance teaching and learning activities in the lab. Based on a suggestion from minority students, in the fall of 1993, the lab was opened for up to 20 hours a week to facilitate independent student practice of assigned nursing procedures; a graduate teaching assistant (master's nursing student) supervised.

A second nursing lab was created specifically in support of the nurse practitioner programs. The lab, known as the Health Assessment Lab (HAL) was on the first floor of Colvard with easy outside access for patients. The lab included two exam rooms equipped for physical assessment, a small reception area, and a records room. The position of coordinator of the Nursing Skills Lab was upgraded to director of Nursing Learning Labs, and Tama Morris, RN, PhD, was appointed as director, following Dr. Sanders's retirement. In planning for the new College of Health and Human Services building, Ms. Morris provided significant leadership in developing several new nursing learning labs for the new building—outfitted with the latest technology for nursing instructio

Advancing Technology in Teaching, Research, and Practice

In 1992, technological advances were changing expectations for nursing education, healthcare delivery, communication, and research nationwide. During the 1990s, the college's strategic goals addressed increasing needs for faculty and students to become knowledgeable about, and to have access to, up-to-date technology. Budgetary resources for technology increased significantly over the next few years.

In the 1992–93 academic year, Mary Curran, RN, PhD, a nursing faculty member, was appointed director of Nursing Informatics Technology to provide leadership in this area. It was only possible to allocate 5% FTE of her time, increasing to 10% in 1993–94, but it was a start. A priority was planning for a Nursing Informatics Learning Lab (NILL). The NILL was wired for multiple computers, and matching funding was obtained from First Data to purchase computers. During the first semester of operation, resources in the lab were limited. NCLEX-RN review materials were purchased and made available in the NILL for student practice, and lab hours were extended two weeks postgraduation to permit BSN students to prepare for the nursing licensing exam. NCLEX-RN testing in North Carolina was computerized for the first time in 1994. Early outcomes included a baseline assessment of faculty computer use and expertise, an inventory of software and hardware in the college, and the availability of consultation to faculty.

A five-year strategic goal was set to purchase a computer for each faculty and staff and to maintain up-to-date technology. By the fall of 1994, the five-year goal was met ahead of schedule with allocations from the CON budget and a $40,000 grant from the university for computer upgrades. Each faculty member had a computer and printer, and a high-quality laser printer was available in each academic department and in a faculty workroom.

At the end of 1994, 15% of undergraduate nursing courses incorporated some instructional software for learning. Faculty enrolled in computer workshops. A graduate research assistant from Computer Science was recruited for a 20% FTE position and allocated to the OSS to help computerize student data for easy access by faculty, tracking of student applications, availability of data for decision-making on admissions, and interface with overall university data.

In the spring of 1994, the CON received approval for additional space in Colvard to establish an audio-visual area for students to study videotapes of nursing procedure simulations. Ruth Mauldin, RN, MSN, prepared numerous audio-visual instructional materials for the lab. An Information Technology Advisory Committee was established with department representatives to provide input on development of a CON plan for information technology. In 1995, CON Strategic Plans for 1996–2001 were developed to guide priorities and allocation of resources, and two elective courses in Nursing Informatics were developed and approved for 1995.

Obtaining university funding for a director of Health Informatics was key to advancing the use of technology. Anne Hakenwerth was recruited in 1995 from Carolinas Medical Center and appointed as the first full-time director of Health Informatics. She led development of the Health Informatics Learning Lab (HILL) for students, assisted the dean and faculty in strategic planning for new technology, chaired the college's Technology Advisory Committee, and established relationships with university computing and technology administrators. She was especially talented in teaching and provided group and individualized instruction to faculty as they developed new online courses.

In 1998, protocols were developed to test the Nightingale Tracker, a hand-held computer introduced to students in undergraduate and graduate courses in community health nursing. The following year, the college would host a national conference on distance education to demonstrate Tracker technology. The conference was attended by 30 nursing faculty from universities in the southern region. The College of Nursing and Health Professions was named by the FITNE Foundation as one of seven Centers of Excellence in Healthcare Technology for nursing programs.

In assessing trends in the delivery of university degree programs, it was noted that the availability of online courses was increasing exponentially each year nationwide, but the availability of online courses at UNC Charlotte was limited. The dean's Technology Innovation Award was established in 1998 to provide summer stipends for faculty interested in increasing their expertise in teaching online courses. All faculty were invited to apply, with priorities given to those who agreed to work on developing a course for the coming year. The director of the Health Informatics Lab was available to provide instruction and individual assistance as the course was developed. Response was enthusiastic as faculty from each department took advantage of this learning opportunity. The Summer Stipend program was offered for three years with positive outcomes as the number of online courses increased.

In 1999, resources were obtained to equip a nursing classroom in Colvard and one in the Belk Gym as smart classrooms with multimedia instruction. That year, as an outcome of enhanced faculty expertise in online instruction, two MSN specialty concentrations were offered in Community Health Nursing and Adult Health Nursing as distance education programs. The School of Nursing was awarded $17,460 in e-learning funding from the UNC Office of the President for distance education in nursing programs.

Serious limitations in physical space in Colvard imposed constraints on how much could be accomplished during the 1990s, yet significant progress ensued. A new building for the College of Health and Human Services, in the design phase in 2002, would include state-of-the-art technologies in multiple smart classrooms, as well as instructional and research labs.

Increasing Support for the College Research Mission

Research to advance nursing science was an important part of the College of Nursing's mission and an expectation for tenure-track appointments. Faculty research productivity was increasingly evaluated in promotion and tenure decisions. Resources to support research were increasing. In accord with this mission, the College of Nursing focused attention on ways to support the nursing research mission.

During the 1992–93 academic year, faculty professional activities included paper and research poster presentations and invitations to address local (9), state (3), regional (2), national (9), and international (3) conferences. Nursing faculty served on the editorial boards of three professional journals, *Advances in Nursing Science,*

Journal of Obstetric, Gynecologic and Neonatal Nursing, and the *Journal of Nurse Midwifery.*

In 1992, a director of Nursing Research position was established, and a faculty member, Ann Newman, RN, PhD, was appointed at 5% FTE to support the research mission. Although this time commitment was limited, it signified the importance of research. A monthly Nursing Research Colloquium was organized for faculty to present ongoing and completed research to peers and to discuss ideas for new directions. Colloquium presentations were announced to the university community, occasionally attracting faculty from other colleges. A profile of faculty clinical and research interests was developed and shared. These activities enhanced awareness of ongoing scholarly work and clinical and research expertise within the College of Nursing. Five faculty members received internal funding for projects from the University Faculty Grants Program. Small grant funding also was obtained from the American Organization of Nurse Executives, Patten Corporation. Elinor Caddell Faculty Scholar Award was established with a generous gift to the College of Nursing from Elinor Caddell, Emeritus Nursing Professor. The award provided funding for faculty pilot projects. The first Elinor Caddell Scholar was awarded in the spring of 1994 to Ann Newman.

Janice Janken, RN, PhD, assumed the role of director of Nursing Research on a 20% FTE basis in the fall of 1993. She represented the College of Nursing in University Research Council meetings and oversaw development of the college's policy and procedures for handling requests for research with students. The Nursing Research Colloquia continued in the CON. A graduate research assistant was appointed and supported 15 nursing faculty members in data entry, bibliographic searches, manuscript preparation, data collection, and analysis. Proposals for external funding significantly increased over the previous year, from 13 proposals (4 were successful) submitted in 1992–93 for $1.9 million to 23 proposals (12 were successful) submitted in 1993–94 for $3.8 million.

In the fall of 1994, the College of Nursing expanded support for research by establishing the college's first Office of Nursing Research under the leadership of a director of Research at 40% FTE. Following the expansion of the College of Nursing to a College of Nursing and Health Professions, this office later became the Office of Research and was administered by an associate dean for Research.

During 1994–95, nine internal grants were submitted to the university from the College of Nursing, and 78% were approved. Another 11 grant proposals were submitted for external funding, and $639,969 was awarded. External funding of grants increased in 1996–97 to $1.2 million. During strategic planning in 1997, College of Nursing and Health Professions research priorities were identified as women's health, chronic illness, promotion of health behavior and lifestyles, community health, health informatics, and geriatric health. That same year, Debra Hymovich, PhD, FAAN, was appointed associate dean for Research and led support for faculty and strengthened relationships with university research committees and administrators until her retirement in 1998. After the first national search for an administrator, Jim McAuley, PhD, an experienced researcher, was recruited from the University of Oklahoma to replace Hymovich.

In the capitol campaign at UNC Charlotte, the College of Nursing had received funding to establish the Dean W. Colvard Distinguished Professor of Nursing Endowed Chair, named in honor of the first chancellor of UNC Charlotte. In 2000, Shirley Travis was named the first Dean W. Colvard Distinguished Professor of Nursing. Dr. Travis developed new linkages in community nursing research and facilitated nursing research teams. That same year, the Federal Division of Nursing gave $591,000 to the MSN program to address state and regional needs.

In 2001, an agreement was formalized between the College of Nursing and Health Professions, New South Health Care Hospice and Palliative Care of Charlotte, and Lincoln County to expand end-of-life research, education, and practice. Initial projects included a study of intimacy at the end of life, and the development of a project to improve patient safety in late-life end-of-life care. Dr. Travis took an active role in this partnership's research. Dean Bishop was also involved as current chair of the Board of Directors of New South Hospice and Palliative Care.

By 2002, two joint manuscripts had been published, and nursing students and social work students were participating in clinical activities.

Also in 2001, a nationally known nursing scholar, Barbara Horowitz, RN, PhD, was appointed as the first A. Sue Kerley Distinguished Visiting Nurse Scholar. Her availability on campus supported ongoing scholarship, and she worked closely with faculty research teams and students, in addition to presenting her research to the university community.

In 2003–04, 38% of faculty submitted proposals for external funding, totaling $9.1 million. Of those proposals, 54% were approved, and $6.4 million was awarded. A proposal to establish a multidisciplinary research center for chronic illness and disability in the College of Health and Human Services was completed and forwarded to UNC Charlotte Provost Joan Lorden, PhD. That year, 73% of all tenure-track faculty in the college published manuscripts, and 70% presented professional papers at national and international conferences.

Growth in Academic Nursing Programs

Academic degree programs available during the 1992–93 academic year included the BSN, RN-BSN Pathways, and MSN degree programs. The MSN program offered five concentrations: Adult Health Nursing, Nursing Administration, Psychiatric Mental Health Nursing, Parent-Child Nursing, and Nurse Anesthesia, which was a collaboration with Carolinas Medical Center (CMC). In the early years of the 2000 decade, a Committee to Plan the PhD in Health Services Research was formed with representatives from each of the departments. This program would be the college's first PhD program.

Undergraduate Programs in Nursing

In the fall of 1992, the newly revised BSN curriculum was implemented, and the first graduates completed the new program in the spring of 1993. Faculty and students praised the new curriculum, emphasizing a more reasonable sequence of courses and improved integration of didactic content and clinical learning experiences. The NC State Board of Nursing and the NLN site visit teams agreed that the new curriculum was strong and the faculty was outstanding and highly qualified. Yet, first writer pass rates on the state licensing exam (NCLEX-RN) were 82%, down from 92% the year before with the old curriculum.

The Undergraduate Curriculum Committee, chaired by Dr. Carveth, conducted an intensive review of the new curriculum and made 12 recommendations to improve NCLEX-RN performance in the future. Noting that the NCLEX-RN was now computerized, several recommendations related to faculty development in computer-assisted instruction (CAI), increasing CAI learning activities in courses, making available the latest NCLEX-RN review materials in the NILL, and expanding open lab hours from 20 to 40 hours a week. All recommendations were implemented by the fall of 1994.

In 1995, strategies to facilitate preparation for the NCLEX-RN exam continued to be strengthened and included: NCLEX-RN review sessions for seniors; purchase of additional NCLEX-RN software available for review in the Health Informatics Lab; integration of NCLEX-RN review in each clinical course; administration of standardized tests in clinical courses; and individual advising of all seniors who scored low on the NLN comprehensive test to assist them in developing strategies for the NCLEX-RN exam. These strategies were effective, and NCLEX-RN pass rates throughout the 1990s met the strategic goal of exceeding 90% pass rates for first writers.

Elective courses for BSN students were approved in 1995: Alcohol Use and Abuse, Teaching the Elderly, Adolescent Health, Critical Thinking in Nursing, and Patient-Centered Care. A paid Clinical Internship course for BSN students was developed and offered on a pilot basis in the summer of 1995 for 15 rising juniors. In 1997, new courses in epidemiology were approved.

In 1994, a review of the RN-BSN Pathways program was completed and recommendations approved by College of Nursing faculty. Recommendations implemented were: increasing the number of faculty teaching in the program; increasing the sequence of courses from two to three semesters to enable students to attend classes two days a week and to facilitate their working in clinical settings. Since there were numerous diploma and associate degree programs in the region, the RN-BSN program was expanded to meet the anticipated demands of students wanting to continue their educations at UNC Charlotte. Approval was granted to offer the RN-BSN program at Rowan Cabarrus Community College and Gaston College in 2000.

The RN-BSN distance education program, developed to meet state and regional needs, had been highly successful. Initial enrollment was strong, and attrition rates were lower than similar programs. Thirty students were admitted to the online program in the fall of 2001, and 24 students graduated in August 2002. Thirty-two students were admitted for the fall of 2002. Funding was received from UNC General Administration to support collaboration with UNC Wilmington to develop an inter-institutional RN-BSN web-based program.

A Health Studies minor for undergraduates was developed and proved popular. Enrollment increased dramatically from eight students in 2002–03 to 60 the following year.

Graduate Programs in Nursing

In 1993–94, planning began in earnest to expand the MSN program to include a Nurse Practitioner concentration, Family Nurse Practitioner (FNP). The FNP curriculum was developed in consultation with Kathy Gillis, RN, PhD, University of California San Francisco, and Cynthia Selleck, RN, PhD, University of South Florida. The FNP program was approved by the university and the College of Nursing in 1995, and the first nurse practitioner students were admitted to the master's program in the 1995–96 academic year.

Two elective courses in Nursing Informatics were developed and approved for the 1994–95 school year. A summer course on Community Health Nursing was offered to regional public health nurses in 1994, with funding from the Public Health

Department. In 1994–95, a cohort of eight students completed the final year of the college's MSN program in Adult Health Nursing in Asheville, with funding from Mountain AHEC.

That same year, registered nurses in the 14-county metropolitan region of Charlotte were surveyed. A high percentage, 77% of the 934 respondents, expressed interest in the MSN program and named Family Nurse Practitioner and Adult Health Nurse Practitioner programs as priorities. A companion survey of employers in the region was mailed to 135 nursing directors, with a 47% response rate. Employers projected a continued need to employ both master's-prepared nurse practitioners and clinical nurse specialists. Data from these surveys were utilized, along with other regional, state, and national reports projecting needs for nurses, to set the college's program priorities.

In 1995, the decision was made to phase out the Parent-Child Nursing MSN concentration due to low student interest, and resources were shifted to the Family Nurse Practitioner (FNP) concentration. The FNP program met a new legislative mandate in North Carolina to prepare critically needed nurse practitioners. A new clinical nurse specialist program was developed in Community Health Nursing (CHN). A grant for the CHN was approved for $531,559 from the Federal Division of Nursing in July 1995. The first students were admitted to the MSN Community Health Nursing program in the fall of 1995. This program prepared advanced practice nurses for leadership roles in community health assessment and planning in rural and urban communities. In 1996, plans were implemented to phase out the Nursing Administration concentration in the MSN program. A dual-degree program in Nursing and Health Administration (MSN/MHA) was approved in 1997.

In 1998, an RN-MSN Early Entry program at Gaston College was approved to meet the need for more nurses with master's degrees in advanced nursing practice. In 2002, the School of Nursing was awarded $17,300 from the Academic Affairs Program Improvement Funds for evaluation of the MSN program. A school nursing track in the MSN program was approved in 2001 to better serve school health needs; the program option was available for graduate students in the MSN program in Community Health Nursing and Family Nurse Practitioner programs. In 2000, MSN specialty concentrations were offered in Community Health Nursing and Adult Health Nursing in a distance education program, and 16 students enrolled.

Planning for the College's First PhD Program

The college's long-range strategic goals included development of PhD programs. In 2003, the increasing resources for research and the availability of researchers in the multidisciplinary College of Health and Human Services suggested the time had arrived. School of Nursing faculty in collaboration with faculty from the Departments of Social Work and Health Behavior and Administration worked on the proposal. The PhD in Health Services Research program, which was approved by the UNC Board of Governors in May 2004, became the first doctoral program in the College of Health and Human Services.

The college's strategic plan was updated with goals for 2003–09 and submitted to Interim Provost Wayne Walcott, PhD, in July 2003. This plan included development of a PhD in Nursing Science, with the Request to Plan targeted for completion in October 2005.

Graduates and Licensing and Certification Exams

In May 1993, 121 BSN students, 15 RN-BSN Pathways students, and 32 MSN students graduated for a total of 168 graduates of the College of Nursing. The commissioning of graduates as military officers was included in the CON's Convocation in 1993. The 1993 graduating senior class presented a silver coffee service as a class gift to the college. The Class of 1994 gave software for the Health Informatics Lab, and in 1995, the class gift was a tree. In 1995, 102 BSN, 58 MSN students, and 17 RN-BSN students completed graduation requirements. In 1996, the first year of the newly organized College of Nursing and Health Professions (CNHP), 725 students graduated from CNHP programs: 106 BSN students, 20 RN-BSN students, 40 MSN students, 26 BS Health Fitness students, and 15 MEd students in Health Promotion. Graduates of undergraduate and graduate programs in the College of Health and Human Services would grow exponentially in the coming years as new programs were developed to meet regional, state, and national needs.

National Certification Exams for MSN Graduates

Graduates of the Nurse Anesthesia MSN program continued to do well each year on the certification exam of the National Association of Nurse Anesthetists, with a consistent 100% pass rate. In 1999, more than half of the graduates achieved a perfect score. Graduates of the Family Nurse Practitioner (FNP) program also achieved pass rates of 100% on national certification exams for both the American Association of Nurse Practitioners (AANP) and the Association of Nurses in Critical Care (ANCC).

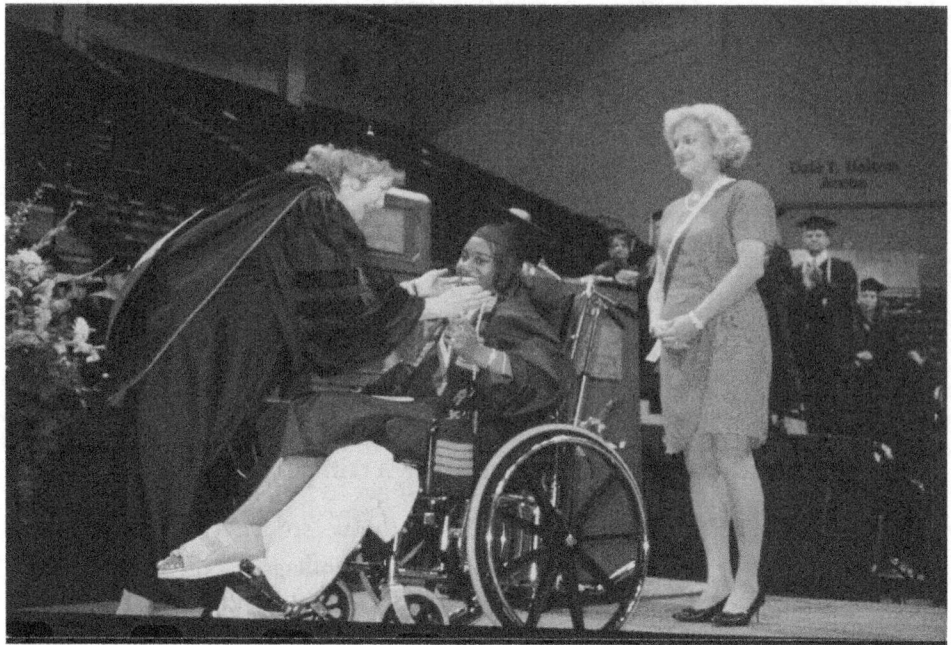

Accidents happen, even to nursing students, but nothing keeps them from graduation.

State Licensing Exam (NCLEX-RN) for BSN Graduates

The 1992 graduates were the last class to complete BSN requirements under the old curriculum. The pass rate on the nursing licensing exam (NCLEX RN) was at 95%. The first writer pass rate on the NCLEX-RN for 1993 BSN graduates was a disappointing 82%, the lowest pass rate in five years; this was the first class to graduate from the new curriculum. Following faculty assessment and development of strategies to assist students, BSN performance began to improve significantly. Key interventions included increasing student time using computerized software in instruction (the NCLEX RN was now computerized) and identifying at-risk students earlier and providing assistance. First writer pass rates for graduates demonstrated the effectiveness of these changes in the 1990s, for example: 95% (1995), 92% (1996), 90% (1997), 92% (1999), 96% (2001).

State and National External Reviews of Nursing Programs

The 1993–94 academic year was characterized by a year of extensive evaluation and highly successful on-site reviews. The North Carolina State Board of Nursing recommended continuing approval of the baccalaureate nursing program and scheduled the next review for 1999.[4] The National League for Nursing (NLN) Board of Review approved the college for the maximum eight years of continuing accreditation and commended the CON and university's commitment to diversity.

The Nurse Anesthesia MSN program completed a successful self-study and on-site review and was awarded continuing accreditation by the American Association of Nurse Anesthetists in the spring of 1997. Accreditation was reaffirmed in 2003.

In 1997, the N.C. State Board of Nursing approved the Family Nurse Practitioner (FNP) program as graduates were meeting state certification to practice as NPs in North Carolina.

The college received preliminary approval in 1998 for BSN and MSN programs from the Commission on Collegiate Nursing Education (CCNE). An on-site review was conducted by a national review team in the fall of 2001, and full CCNE accreditation was awarded for BSN and MSN programs. (The decision had been made to seek accreditation from the CCNE in 2001, a growing trend in collegiate nursing education, rather than reaccreditation from NLN in 2002.)

The college completed an application for its multidisciplinary MHA in Health Administration program (with a dual-degree MHA/MSN option) and submitted it to the Accrediting Commission Education for Health Services Administration (ACEHSA) in the spring of 2004. Other initiatives seeking accreditation included: Social Work, Health Administration, Athletic Training, and a Rock Climbing program. Engaging in accreditation activities was becoming a cottage industry in the College of Health and Human Services. All programs were accredited.

Study Abroad Programs in Health Care

In the summer of 1995, Dean Bishop initiated the exploration of study abroad programs for students focused on nursing care and healthcare systems in other countries. The first program to be offered was a summer program to study healthcare delivery systems and healthcare issues in Holland, France, Belgium, and Germany. Arrangements were made for healthcare providers in each country's clinical sites (e.g., hospitals, nursing homes, clinics, community centers) to provide instruction and tours. A nursing faculty member traveled with the students to provide support and instruction. New faculty were brought into the program every two years to introduce faculty to the merits of studying abroad and to broaden awareness of cultural issues in health care in other countries.

Two groups participated in the European Study Abroad Program in 1998. Eleven senior nursing students visited healthcare systems in Holland, Germany, and Belgium; and a second group of 44 health professions students and public school teachers traveled to Maastricht to participate in a comparative study of U.S. and Holland public policies related to sexuality and sex education.

The program was cancelled for the 2002 academic year due to low enrollment following the September 11th tragedy at the World Trade Center; the program resumed the next year. In 2004, the European Summer Study Abroad program focused on a Comparative Study of National Healthcare Systems in Western Europe and the United States.

A gift from the Alice and John Harney family established an endowment to support international travel scholarships for students in the college. The first Harney Scholar was appointed in 1998. By 2004, seven students had received scholarships to study abroad.

In 1998, the college hosted its first international visiting professor. Laila Farhood, RN, PhD, professor of nursing and medicine, from the American University of Beirut, Lebanon, was appointed for the spring and summer semesters as the Visiting Dean W. Colvard Distinguished Professor of Nursing. Dr. Farhood presented lectures in graduate and undergraduate courses and taught a graduate course focused on family health and intervention. She also presented her research on stress in families in areas of violence and war in the Middle East.

Faculty and Teaching Excellence

There were 39 nursing faculty in the College of Nursing in 1993–94 (including the dean), 34 were full-time and five were part-time; Eighty-seven percent of full-time faculty were in tenure-track positions, and 48% had achieved tenure. The percentage of faculty with doctoral degrees was 70%. Clinical expertise in nursing specialties included: adult health nursing, pediatric nursing, neonatal nursing, obstetric nursing, community health nursing, nursing informatics, and nursing administration. Four faculty members had completed national certification: pediatric nurse practitioner (Elaine Nishioka); RN, MSN, ANA clinical specialist in adult psychiatric nursing (Carolyn Maynard, RN, PhD); and ANCC nurse practitioners (Emily Chiles, RN, MSN, and Marilyn Smith, RN, MSN). By 1995, four nursing faculty had been elected as Fellows in the American Academy of Nursing (FAAN) for contributions to nursing and health care (Dean Sue Bishop, RN, PhD, Barbara Carper, RN, PhD, Sara Torres, RN, PhD, and Debra Hymovich, RN, PhD). By 2000, nursing faculty in the School of Nursing included four faculty members who were certified as family nurse practitioners (Carolyn Maynard, Mary Curran, and Kay Boggs) and an adult health nurse practitioner (Linda Steele).

In the 1990s, the need for nurse practitioners was great and growing. In response, the college developed the first nurse practitioner master's program, with plans to offer the Family Nurse Practitioner (FNP) concentration as the first NP program. While the need to prepare nurse practitioners was great, there was a critical shortage of nurse practitioner faculty. This limited the ability of colleges to expand NP programs to meet projected needs. The College of Nursing and Health Professions was fortunate to obtain funding from a new initiative by the Kellogg Foundation for the preparation of nurse practitioner faculty. Kellogg FNP faculty fellowships were awarded to three tenure-track faculty members in 1996–97 for a year of intensive, full-time study as nurse practitioners, in out-of-state university programs: Kay Boggs, RN, PhD, Carolyn Maynard, RN, PhD, and Mary Curran, RN, PhD (one faculty member from each of the three academic departments in nursing). In their absence, additional part-time faculty were employed to assist with teaching. The recruitment of Linda Steele, RN, PhD, adult nurse practitioner, added significantly to the cadre of faculty who were now prepared to provide instruction in nurse practitioner programs.

Nursing faculty were engaged in interdisciplinary relationships within the university to a limited degree in 1993–94 (e.g., a joint research project on the design of nursing homes with Bettie Glenn, RN, PhD, and Randy Swanson, PhD, from the Department of Architecture and a collaboration with Brocker Health Center on a Health Fair for university students. A nursing course on HIV Infection and AIDS was open to university students. Several faculty held joint appointments in the College of Arts and Sciences and made contributions to women's health studies and gerontology. Interdisciplinary courses continued to be developed by nursing faculty as electives for university students. Strategic planning during the 1990s, resulting in the creation of a multidisciplinary College of Health and Human Services, had created new opportunities for multidisciplinary relationships to develop in teaching and research. The proposed interdepartmental PhD in Health Services Research in 2004 is one example. The coming years are rich with possibility.

Nursing faculty have historically been active in serving on university task forces and committees. In 1993, they were members of 26 university committees and task forces. These activities continued through the 1990s and into the early 2000s, with nursing faculty assuming leadership roles in university service, such as: Dr. Carper, who was co-chair of the Health Issues Academy, Dr. Newman who was secretary and president of the University Faculty Council, Dean Bishop who was co-chair of the Health Commission and chair of the Ad Hoc Committee to Evaluate and Revise the University Strategic Plan.

Nursing faculty continued to be active at the local, state, regional, and national levels and assumed many national leadership positions, such as: president, National

Association of Hispanic Nurses; president, International Consortium of Parse Scholars; member of the American Nurses Association Council on Cultural Diversity; president, Society for Research and Education in Psychiatric Mental Health Nursing; member of the Research Grants Review Committees, National Institute of Mental Health (NIMH). Dean Bishop, Dr. D'Antonio, and Dr. Torres were active in accreditation reviews of nursing programs in other universities, serving as consultants for the National League for Nursing (NLN); and Dr. Newman was elected to the N.C. Board of Nursing.

The University of the State of New York (SUNY) awarded the Carry Lenberg Distinguished Alumnus Award to Dr. Cody in 1996. Dean Bishop was awarded the Distinguished Alumni Award from the Indiana University School of Education Alumni Association in 2000.

Faculty Teaching Excellence

Excellence in teaching has always been a core component of the College of Nursing, and multiple mechanisms have been in place to evaluate the nursing programs and courses, including student evaluations, as a routine part of the assessment process. In response to a mandate from UNC General Administration, the College of Nursing developed guidelines and procedures for the reviews. The guidelines were approved by the CON Faculty Organization and Provost and Vice Chancellor Dubois for implementation in the 1994–95 academic year. Student evaluations were conducted for each course and were a component of annual faculty reviews of faculty. Faculty evaluated department chairs and the dean. The dean's evaluation was conducted by the College Review Committee.

A college that values teaching effectiveness will recognize teaching excellence. During the 1990s, three teaching awards were developed in the College of Nursing (and College of Nursing and Health Promotion) to acknowledge dedicated and creative teachers. In the spring of 1993, the Undergraduate Teaching Excellence Award was established to recognize excellence in teaching baccalaureate students. Recipients of the Undergraduate Teaching Excellence Award were Dr. Judith Carveth (1994), Professor Carol Fray (1995), Dr. Ann Newman (1996), Dr. Linda Johanson (2001), Linda Probst (2002), and Dr. Alan Young (2004). The Graduate Teaching Excellence Award was established in 1994, and the first recipient was Dr. Linda Moore. The Graduate Teaching Excellence Award was presented to Dr. Bettie Glenn in 1995, Dr. Linda Berne in 1996, Tim Lightfoot in 2001, and Dr. Carole Winston in 2004. A teaching award to recognize excellence in clinical teaching was established, and the first recipient of the Clinical Teaching Excellence Award was Dr. Delores Sanders in 1999 and Tama Morris in 2004. Faculty receiving the

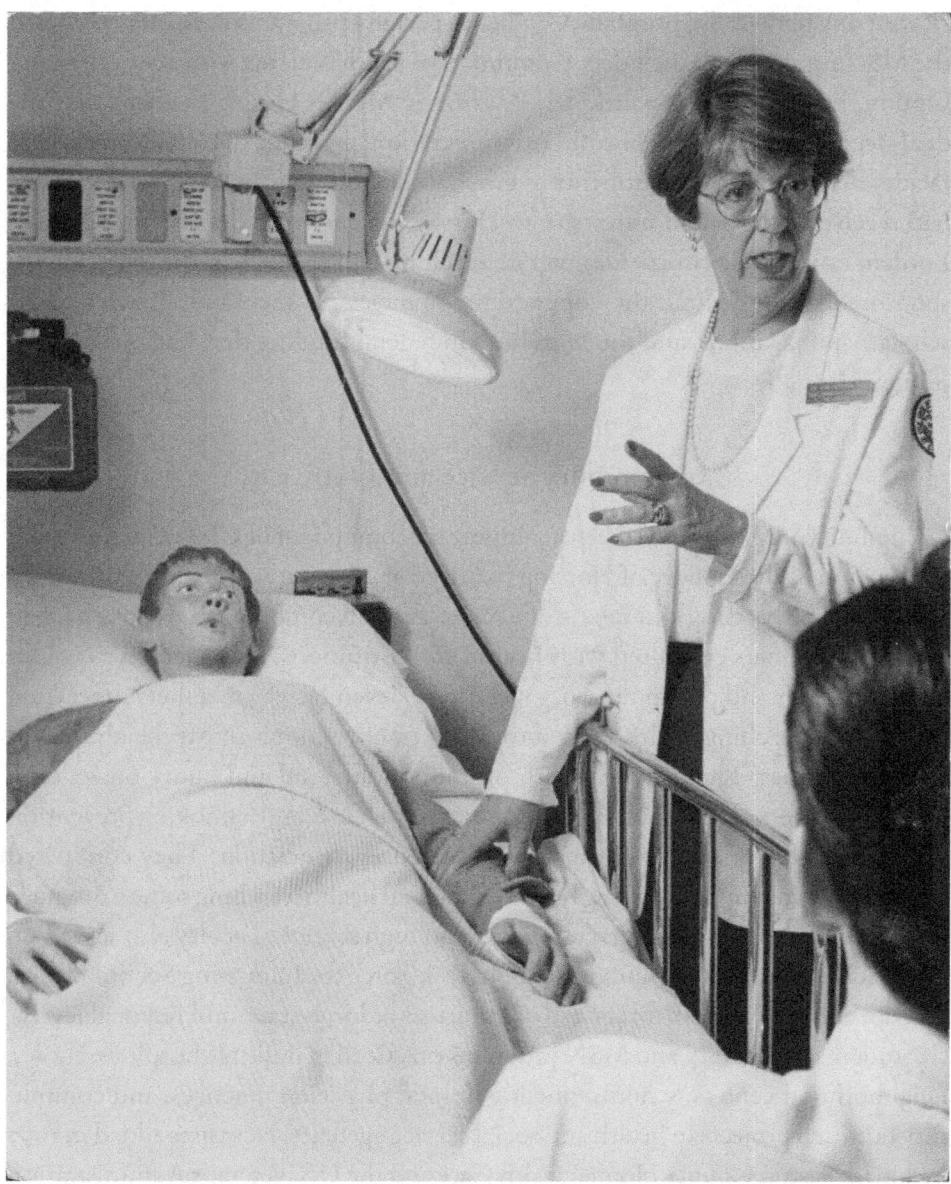

Ann Newman, Bank of America Award recipient.

annual college teaching awards were announced at the annual CON convocation in May. Two faculty were recipients of the university's Nations Bank Award for Teaching Excellence and the UNC Board of Governors Award for Teaching—Dr. Ann Newman in 1996 and Dr. Linda Berne in 2002.

In 2003, the Department of Family and Community Nursing captured the UNC Charlotte Provost's Award for Excellence in Teaching. This department's faculty taught community health, psychiatric mental health, pediatrics, and obstetrics nursing in the BSN program. Graduate specialty programs were offered within the MSN program and included: Community Health Nursing with a School Nurse Option, Family Nurse Practitioner, Psychiatric Mental Health Nursing, and the dual-degree Nursing and Health Administration program (MHA/MSN). Five faculty held adjunct appointments in other academic departments. Several faculty had received college and university teaching excellence awards. The provost, Dr. Lorden, noted their efforts to integrate teaching and practice in the department-sponsored nursing clinic they operate for homeless women and children, their scholarly publications, and the $1 million in federal funding they had received for program initiatives.

Community Service and Outreach

Community Service has also been an important component of UNC Charlotte and the mission of the College of Nursing (College of Nursing and Health Professions and School of Nursing). In 1994, 11 faculty served on community advisory boards, 9 faculty members consulted with healthcare institutions, and 3 served as volunteers at schools and community organizations. Seven faculty members supervised 215 students teaching health-related topics at public schools in Mecklenburg and Gaston counties. They taught health promotion, first aid and injury prevention, HIV prevention, alcohol abuse prevention, seat belt use, and a smoking prevention project in collaboration with the American Lung Association. They conducted health screenings to assess eating habits and dental health, reaching some 7,610 public school students in elementary, middle, and high schools. Faculty also served on the Mecklenburg County Public Schools Task Force for Improving School Health and dozens of other task forces and committees at local, state, and regional levels.

Students in the BSN and MSN programs practiced in multiple hospitals, clinics, neighborhood centers, schools, nursing homes, physician practices, and community outreach projects in health and social service agencies. New sites added in 1992 included Gaston County Home Health Care and the U.S. Veterans Administration Hospital in Salisbury. Students practiced in 21 community agencies in 1994, and additional sites continued to be added each year.

Likewise, student involvement in community service activities increased significantly during the 1990s. By 2004, 100% of all baccalaureate and master's programs in the college included community service learning activities.

In 1994, academic departments began to consider supporting a departmental community service project. The Department of Community Health, Psychiatric Mental Health Nursing and Nursing Systems adopted the Nursing Clinic for

Homeless Women and Children as a department project. This clinic was managed and staffed by volunteer CON faculty and students in space provided by the Salvation Army. In 1994, the clinic was renamed the Nursing Center for Health Promotion and continued to operate under the leadership of Dr. Cody. An annual walk-a-thon raised $3,290 for the center that year, which saw a total of 510 visits from women and children. External funding was obtained to offer an HIV-prevention project at the center, and instruction was a collaborative effort between nursing and social work faculty. In 1998, the Sisters of Mercy Foundation awarded $93,000 to support center services.

The Department of Parent-Child and Women's Health Nursing partnered with Garinger High School (a health magnet school with more than 50% minority students) to explore preparation of high school students for health careers.

In partnership with the Carolinas Piedmont Alzheimer's Association, MSN students in Community Health Nursing completed a two-county assessment of caregiver needs under the supervision of Dr. David Langford, RN, PhD. The report was presented by students at the association's annual meeting. In 2002, students conducted two health fairs, one at the Salvation Army for Homeless Women and Children and one at a local high school. Community service continues to be a strong commitment in nursing programs, and faculty are active in a variety of agencies, hospitals, centers, clinics, and community-based programs and schools as consultants, teachers, practitioners, and board members. A 2001 survey of the college's faculty and administrators found that 97% were actively engaged in community service activities.

Leadership for Continuing Education

A director of Continuing Education (Dr. Linda Moore) was appointed in 1992 for a 10% FTE to oversee the development of long-range plans in continuing education. The first goal was to offer the minimum number of programs that would qualify the College of Nursing to apply for Continuing Education (CE) provider status from the North Carolina Nurses Association. This goal was achieved by the spring of 1993, when three CE programs were attended by almost 350 nurses.

In 1994, a survey of nurses in 13 counties surrounding the Charlotte metropolitan region demonstrated high interest in CE programming in nursing, including courses on immunodeficient diagnoses, critical care nursing, and cardiac care nursing. The demands are expected to increase. The School of Nursing is poised to make a unique contribution in this area, given the expertise of its faculty.

The college's director of Continuing Education continued as a 20% FTE ap-

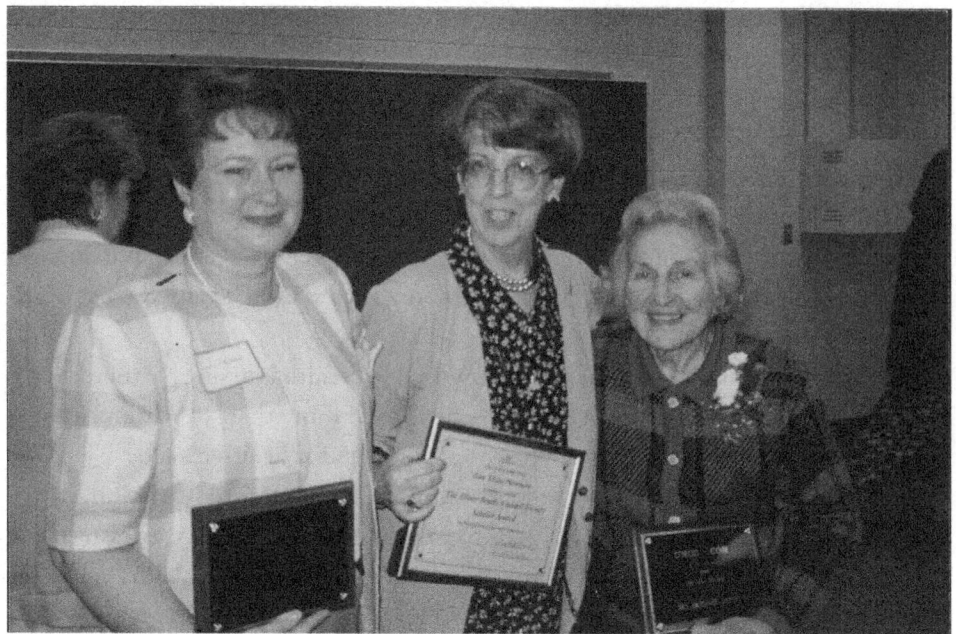

Nancy Mathias receives Alumni Award; Ann Newman receives the first Elinor Brooks
Caddell Faculty Award; Miss Bonnie, always a cheerleader for nursing, 1994.

pointment in 1994–95. A Community CE Advisory Committee was established
to assist with long-range planning. During the College of Nursing's Annual Spring
Lecture, the first Distinguished Service Award was presented to Bonnie Cone. Miss
Bonnie, as she was affectionately known, was the founder of UNC Charlotte. In
1996, the award went to Professor Emerita Elinor Caddell.

In 1997, the first Distinguished Alumni Award was presented to Nancy Mathias,
and in 1998 the award was presented to Agnes Weisiger, MSN, NP, and Judith
Grubbs, RN, MSN.

In 1999, continuing education programs were offered for 410 health professionals in the state and region. Co-sponsors included the Metrolina Association of Diabetes Educators, Charlotte Chapter of Rehabilitation Nurses, and the Southeastern
Chapter of the International Consortium of Parse Scholars.

CPR training for certification continued to be offered by nursing faculty each
year for all college faculty, and in 2000, the library staff. In 2001, a workshop on
publishing was attended by 30 faculty and professional staff from UNC Charlotte,
Queens College, Winthrop College, and three area healthcare institutions.

Continuing education offerings reflected an increased emphasis on nursing research as did the development of an Annual Nursing Research Conference. In 1999,

104 nurse researchers from six southern states participated in the college's fourth annual Nursing Research Conference, focused on Research in Women's Health. In 2001, 118 health professionals from five states attended the fifth annual Nursing Research Symposium on integrative health practices.

Renovating Space and Designing a New Building

By 1992, the College of Nursing was quickly outgrowing the first floor of the Colvard Building. Resources were allocated to upgrade facilities, erect temporary walls, and re-allocate space. The dean commented on the need for a new building frequently in university meetings.

During 1992–93, renovations in Colvard created a new 50-seat classroom, a seminar/meeting room, and a department chair's office. The university fixed a problem with mold on an exterior wall, and the interior got much-needed paint and new carpeting.

Two offices and a reception area adjacent to the college's central administration, which had been loaned in the 1980s to the university, were returned to the college for the centralized Office of Student Services. Two conference rooms were partitioned to create faculty offices. An additional request to University Academic Affairs resulted in the return of a reception area and two offices in Colvard to establish the Office of Nursing Research.

In 2000, funds were obtained to renovate space in the Colvard Building to create the Advanced Health Assessment Lab (HAL). The lab was constructed with a reception area and separate exam rooms for physical assessments. As the twenty-first century approached, the college had run out of creative solutions to find space for the continued growth of nursing programs.

In 2002, following several proposals by local architectural firms, the PEASE Engineering and Architecture Firm was selected by Chancellor Woodward to design a new academic building for the College of Health and Human Services (CHHS). The firm selected was the only one that sent architects to meet with the dean and faculty to solicit ideas prior to delivering its proposal, and this was considered an indicator of the collaboration that might occur during the building design.

A series of meetings were held with the design team—Gary Runyan (architect), Debbie Barger (design), and John Duncan (PEASE architect and administrator)—to create a shared understanding of projected needs for the College of Health and Human Services. An ad hoc committee was established with representatives from academic departments, administrators, and directors to provide input in the design of the building. Dean Bishop and the other co-chairs of the University Health Commission (Dean Bob Mundt and Dr. Bill Brandon) visited the multidisciplinary College of Health Sciences building at the University of Central Florida, and Dean Bishop and the Nursing Skills director, Dr. Tama Morris, RN, traveled with two members of the architectural team to tour the College of Nursing building at the University of Maryland, specifically to review the nursing labs. These visits were most helpful in identifying best practices in building design, as well as aspects of the designs to avoid.

A sample of the assumptions that evolved as guidelines in the planning included: (1) a cluster arrangement of faculty offices to foster collaboration, with departmental offices and central administration on the fourth floor; (2) a conference room for each academic department and a faculty-staff lounge on each floor; (3) a first-floor Office of Student Services for easy access; (4) a larger space for the Health Informatics Lab, group rooms for student computer projects, and administrative offices and space for graduate assistants; (5) a group of learning labs and classrooms on the same floor, interview rooms with one-way glass for research and teaching, and advanced practice nursing labs; and (6) an auditorium on the first floor for large classes and access to kitchen facilities for receptions.

There were multiple buildings in various stages of approval and construction on campus during the 1990s and 2000s. Chancellor Woodward had specific expectations for how all the new buildings would complement one another to create a timeless appearance of the UNC Charlotte campus. All the new buildings were brick with a traditional design. A lengthy discussion about the proposed cupola[5] for the CHHS building ensued in one meeting with Chancellor Woodward, Dean Bishop, and the architects. The chancellor wasn't sold on the idea, but a comment from one of the architects sealed the deal. "This building is in the center of campus," he said, "and the cupola on the building creates the appearance of a university campus." When the building was completed, there were compliments all around for the cupola. Many photos of the UNC Charlotte campus on brochures and programs include the CHHS building and its cupola.

The building design was completed, construction was bid, and a builder was selected to begin construction in June 2004. Dean Bishop retired on July 1, 2004.

My Tenure

My tenure as dean at UNC Charlotte occurred during a period of fast-paced and dramatic changes. During these 12 years, the structure of the College of Nursing was transformed to a College of Nursing and Health Professions and then a College of Health and Human Services, with a new School of Nursing in a multidisciplinary college.

At times, I felt like an air traffic controller at a busy airport with projects and issues landing and taking off at warp speed. There is no doubt that the strategic planning process was the engine that stimulated change and guided our growth. All the efforts to develop outcome evaluation procedures for continued assessment of programs, services, faculty, and administrators gave useful data to aid decision-making. As the college grew, preparing for accreditation self-studies and on-site visits became a job unto itself.

Planning the new building was an exciting venture. I was surprised and honored that the university named the CHHS Auditorium for me. When I returned to campus for the dedication, I remember standing in the dean's office with John Duncan, the PEASE architect, just the two of us, looking out the window at the campus. "I've designed a lot of buildings in my career," Duncan said, "but this building is one of the ones I am most proud of designing."

My greatest pleasure over the years was the opportunity to work with talented and dedicated faculty in the college, from all disciplines. They were simply outstanding! While the work was demanding, there were so many times when someone created a social event to create a laugh or welcome break in the day. On Halloween, clowns, rock musicians, and witches conducted business as usual. One Christmas season, two empty baskets were set up in the college, and faculty were invited to share samples of their cooking and baking as gifts for Chancellor Woodward and Provost Dubois; the baskets were filled to the brim with cookies, treats, and even homemade hot fudge sauce. Another December, a door decorating contest was proposed by one of the nursing faculty. Chancellor Emeritus Dean Colvard and Mrs. Colvard agreed to select the winner. Every December, a holiday reception was held at the dean's home for faculty, donors, and faculty and administrators from other departments.

The nursing students had their own fun too. They planned a raffle to raise money at the senior picnic at Reedy Creek Park one year. For each dollar donated, the benefactor got a vote for a college faculty member to kiss a pig. Yes, the pig was real, and yes, I did. I wondered how many dollars faculty members put in the jar to make me the winner. Hmmm.

The university administrators I had the privilege to work with set a high bar for excellence and leadership. So many were open to collaboration and provided support for strategic growth. In particular, collegial relationships with Chancellor Woodward, Vice Chancellor and Provost Dubois, and deans of the graduate school and other academic colleges were much valued. I mentioned to a colleague in another university once that UNC Charlotte was very open to new ideas. "You take an idea to someone to consider," I said, "and the response right away is, 'Let's discuss

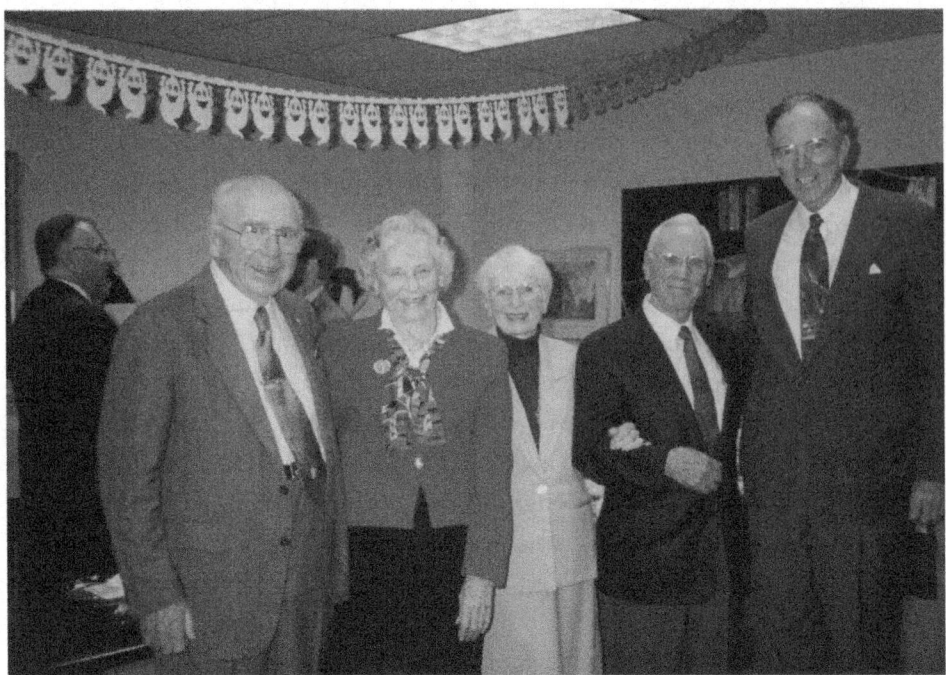

Chancellor Dean, Martha Colvard, and Chancellor E. K. Fretwell attend our celebration.

it.'" UNC Charlotte is unique in that it has never suffered from mismanagement.

It was a privilege to know the retired university founder, Bonnie Cone. I can see Miss Bonnie in her advanced years, sitting at a reception with a group of enthralled students. Dr. Cone attended the College of Nursing's Annual Spring Luncheon without fail, for many years. I learned much from discussions with Chancellor Emeritus Fretwell and Chancellor Emeritus Colvard about the history of the university and about the leadership they provided during their tenures as chancellor. Chancellor Emeritus Colvard remained involved in the College of Nursing for several years. It was a personal and professional privilege to know him.

When the faculty and administrators began the procession for the 2000 Convocation of the College of Nursing and Health Professions, the musicians began to play the theme from *2001: A Space Odyssey*. As I proudly led the faculty into the arena and onto the stage, I was struck by so many new beginnings—the transition to a new College of Health and Human Services with a School of Nursing, new strategic goals, a new century.

Faculty Scrapbook

These remembrance stories were written as a request from Dr. Bill Cody who was chair of the Department of Family and Community Nursing. He used this strategy of storytelling for faculty to get to know each other better and to celebrate the good things and accomplishments from the College of Nursing/College of Nursing and Health Professions.

YVONNE YOUSEY

A Night to Remember[6]

The terrible night had passed. It had been every woman's, or perhaps every person's, worst nightmare. While sleeping alone, a persistent noise from the window awakened me and I stood up to check it out. A large dark form was suddenly in the room lunging at me and I began fighting for my life as it flashed before me. I fought and slid from his grasp, and fought again and escaped. I ran to the door to make noise and as I did, he fled into the dark night. The event was over in probably less than thirty seconds although it seemed like a lifetime. I was not physically harmed. The next few hours were a blur of detectives, police, and paramedics hovering—taking depositions, presenting me with lineups of possible perpetrators, asking questions, getting information. Then it was over as the dawn appeared in the eastern sky. I began the task of determining the meaning of it all.

My aim is not to dwell on the negative and frightening aspects of this experience, but to remember those who stood or walked by my side as the healing process began. Not the least of these were my coworkers and the students at UNC Charlotte. As I walked into school the next day, there were hugs from Carolyn, Pam, Michelle, and others. Kathy, in her eternal wisdom and kindness, came to the door of my office and said, "I can't believe that this happened. You are my hero." Others listed to my story again and again, told me how brave I was, and asked how they could help.

Four days later, I walked into the graduate research class I was teaching. The weekend had been difficult and I felt unprepared for class. Thirty-four students waited for me. As I entered the classroom, a student approached me with a question. Almost before she could get the question out, she looked at me and said, "Are you okay?" in such a way that I wondered how she could know. I responded to her question and then said, "How did you know?" She answered by saying that she could see it in my face. After I explained the recent events, she said, "Yes, I know, and I have my own story." Class began and I never heard the story.

The students listened quietly, slightly aghast, as I briefly shared my story. We got through the class that night and when I arrived home, the telephone was ringing. It rang several more times that night—at the other end were students who were concerned enough to call to say they cared and some to share their own stores. The next evening at the end of class, a card appeared on my desk. In it were kind and caring words from each and every one of my students. These were students who had no obligation to care for me. Their willingness to be supportive, caring individuals made the road to healing a little easier during these days. I shall never forget them.

I was impressed and deeply grateful for the caring and concern of my colleagues and the students at UNC Charlotte during this experience. None of us would ask for an experience such as this. Nor did I. Out of it came a new appreciation for those who surround me, especially the wonderful people at UNC Charlotte and students with whom I have the privilege of working.

YVONNE YOUSEY, UPDATE 2017[7]

Eleven years have passed since the events leading to this story occurred and nine years have passed since I left UNC Charlotte School of Nursing. Fortunately, the negative memories have become a blur and the positive ones of supportive colleagues and students remain more clearly in my mind.

A recent visit to campus made me realize how UNC Charlotte has changed. Colvard Hall, previous home to the School of Nursing, now houses a Research Institute and the School of Nursing is located on what seems to be the other side of an ever-growing campus. The rhythms of time and change continue—through it all I remember the privilege of teaching at UNC Charlotte. My skills as a nurse educator fit the needs of the School of Nursing and the two meshed to create a wonderfully positive experience for me. Relationships with students and faculty enriched my life and resulted in the three years at UNC Charlotte being the highlight of my teaching career. Social media has allowed me to keep in touch with many of these wonderful people, and it is reassuring to see the contributions they continue to make to the nursing profession.

I returned to Colorado when I left UNC Charlotte after three years and continued my teaching career for another eight years at UNC (University of Northern Colorado) in Greeley. During this time, I occasionally saw faculty colleagues from UNC Charlotte at conferences and enjoyed these special times of connection. I am now semi-retired and continue a part-time primary care clinical practice in pediatrics. That allows time to enjoy my two grandsons, to travel, and do those things in life that full-time jobs do not allow.

My tenure at UNC Charlotte was relatively brief and my memories of the history of the School of Nursing are somewhat elusive. I never personally knew Bonnie Cone, Edith Brocker, Elinor Caddell, and others who nurtured the school through its early days, establishing the solid foundation for growth to its current status. I appreciate the commitment, dedication, and contributions of these founding women and nursing leaders who have followed and am grateful that I could share in the education of professional nurses at UNC Charlotte.

TAMA MORRIS[8]

The School of Nursing and Hope

When I think of the School of Nursing. I think of the word *hope. Hope* is tied into so many aspects of our daily life at the school. In August, we have the *hope* that each incoming class will be the best of the best. We *hope* that they will learn from us and we will learn from them. The students come to us with the *hope* of a strong education that will lead to a bright, productive and worthwhile future.

We also *hope* that the new faculty member is just what we need! I am afraid there are times we forget to *hope* that we are just what they need. We *hope* that this one will be the one with the answers to our brain that seems to have few ideas left and our "to do" list that seems to have too many things left on it. The new faculty come to us with the *hope* of growing a career and the *hope* of belonging. They *hope* to make a difference.

In May, as our students go forth in the world, we *hope* that they will pass NCLEX and certification exams. We *hope* that they will gain employment and we *hope* that they will make us proud. This is probably one of the times our *hope* and that of our students is aligned.

And I think we secretly have one more *hope* . . . *hope* that the summer will be just a little bit longer this year. *Hope* that we will return renewed and refreshed as we again get a new class and new faculty for our Circle of Hope.

TAMA MORRIS, UPDATE 2017

As an update, my career has progressed and reflecting now as a dean, I would say that I continue to have the same hope for nursing education. The beauty of working in academia is that we live in cycles and each one begins with new hope.

The hope I would add is to hear from our graduates and colleagues as their hopes become reality. There is nothing better than connecting with a former student and learning where nursing has taken them or watching the career of a faculty member grow.

BILL CODY[9]

The Day Barbara Carper hired Bill Cody at UNC Charlotte

It was spring 1992 and I was "ABD" in my doctoral program at the University of South Carolina, busily collecting data. I had spent two years studying continental European philosophy and phenomenology driving back and forth between Charlotte and Columbia to attend to my doctoral classes and trying to turn myself into a community-based, family-centered nurse after 12 years of hospital nursing, mostly in ICUs and similar settings. I was devoting most of my time in my doctoral studies to building on the knowledge base that I had begun in New York studying under Rosemarie Parse. I had made it my mission to understand the roots of her theory as well as humanly possible. This required an immersion in literature beyond anything I had experienced before. I had a great mentor for community health in my dissertation chair, Pam Clarke, but still had very little experience, having just moved my practice into home health care within the past year. I was accepting limited home visits with my time dominated by my push to get through the dissertation as quickly as possible. I still did not have a very clear idea of what my postdoctoral career would look like.

There was an ad in the *Charlotte Observer* for a full-time lecturer in Community Health Nursing at the University of North Carolina at Charlotte. I had been a part-time lecturer in Adult Health Nursing at Hunter College in New York and being "ABD," I figured I had a chance at this position, despite my limited background in community health nursing, so I sent my CV. A few weeks later, I was about to give up hope on the position, when Barbara Carper called me and asked if I would like to come in for an interview. Barbara Carper is the most commonly cited author by far in the area of nursing scholarship in which I do most of my work, and it turned out she was serving as interim dean at UNC Charlotte. This was impressive. I began to get excited about the possibility of joining the faculty at UNC Charlotte. I am basically from Charlotte, with memories dating back to age eight in the early sixties, when it was a sleepy small city where an eight-year-old could take the city bus by himself downtown. UNC Charlotte is really the only place for a bona fide nursing scholar to make a career in Charlotte. So I was extremely pleased to think that I might be able to continue my career there by way of this job. I was now set to interview with Barber Carper.

The day of my interview came. That was my first experience of the Colvard North building. Barbara's office was in the center office in Adult Health Nursing that later became Linda Moore's. By this time it was summer and there weren't many faculty around. The College of Nursing seemed a rather sleepy and pleasant place and everyone I met was very cordial. The part of the interview I remember best was when Barbara noted that we were both smokers, we could have our interview down by the lake and have a little smoke together. I remember sitting together on a bench by the edge of the lake and talking about nursing philosophy and theory. I shared with Barbara that it was my belief that nursing would only come into its own as an academic discipline when nursing practice and research came to be guided by nursing theories. To my delight, Barbara just calmly said that she believed that too, as if every rationale nurse would. . . . I knew then that if I were offered the position I would take it.

That fall I learned just how much I did not yet know about community health nursing. I learned that Barbara Carper was not apparently as interested as an administrator in the four ways of knowing that she had written about so eloquently. I learned more about departmental politics as I struggled to keep my head above water with colleagues in Community Health Nursing who didn't really trust me, seeing me as an interloper who was not "really" community health and had these wild ideas about theory and qualitative research. Later, I learned just how very lucky I was to get the position and to what extent the stars had had to be in the right positions for things to turn out the way they did. I finished my dissertation that academic year and was greeted upon my return to the UNC campus with a truly generous celebration. The opportunity came to apply for a tenure-track position. I did, and, thankfully, I was offered the position . . . which led to my serving for 12 years and counting on the faculty at UNC Charlotte. At least I think now I am beginning to be accepted as a community health nurse.

Update provided by Bill Cody, September 2017[10]

My years at UNC Charlotte were among the most rewarding of my career. My co-workers were truly wonderful, and I was proud of what the School of Nursing and the Department of Family and Community Nursing accomplished. It was a happy 13 years for me in a way that was never matched in my later career, although I had some successes. I went on to become dean of the School of Nursing and founding dean of the Blair College of Health at Queens University of Charlotte, where we started the first Clinical Nurse Leader program in North Carolina. After that, I moved to Chicago to serve as director of the graduate-level-only DePaul University School of Nursing, where I had the privilege to serve as we opened the Doctor of Nursing Practice program and a remote campus in North Chicago. My last executive role was with Chamberlain College of Nursing serving as campus president—in Atlanta. Now in 2017, at age 62, I am taking a break from full-time work to pursue a long-held interest of mine and to undertake a master of arts in Peace Studies from the University for Peace, a global university for peace created by the United Nations. In my mind there is a thread with that theme stretching all the way back to my first day at UNC Charlotte. I am grateful for the years I spent at UNC Charlotte and happy for the advances that the School of Nursing and the university have made in the ensuing years.

PEGGY PATTON[11]

My Story

When I was anticipating moving from Albany, New York, to Charlotte, I interviewed in several different situations for a job that I would enjoy and one where I could feel challenged. The job that I was leaving in the New York State Education Department was one that I really enjoyed and was the type of job that I had worked toward for much of my professional career. It was a hard job to leave and even harder to replace, for enjoyment reasons and for economic reasons. At the time that we made the move here from New York, we had four children in college. One of the places I interviewed was UNC Charlotte in the College of Nursing and Health Professions. I was interviewed by Dr. Jan Janken. Dean Bishop called and offered me a one-year appointment as a lecturer, at a rather meager salary. Because of the expensive output I had with four children in college, I said "No, thank you." The dean commented that she hated to let me go because I had a Clinical Specialty in Community Health, which apparently was a little hard to find. She also told me that she would put me in an agency relatively near my house. I declined the job.

I actually made the move down here in 1993 and took a job in home health. From then until 1999, I did home health in one form or another. I worked for a government agency, for two agencies owned by a single person, to agencies owned by a publicly traded, large for-profit organization. I worked as a clinical nurse specialist, a nurse educator, a director of clinical operations, and lastly as an agency director. I was working at the agency where Dean Bishop had said she would send me for my clinical interacting with students when I met the new instructor from UNC Charlotte. His name was Bill Cody. We had nice conversations about New York City because he had lived and worked there for many years and had done his master's degree there at one of the City University of New York campuses. I was homesick and his conversations about New York made me feel much better. He was continuing his education at USC when I knew him.

Nearly seven years later, as a home health agency director, I was getting very tired of "fighting" with Medicare, because I was determined to get paid for every patient we cared for. Furthermore, the national company who owned us was beginning to shut down agencies all across the country that were not making money. When the viable agencies belonging to this company dropped from 22 to 4, I decided that I really did not need this kind of a pressure job anymore. I resigned, and about two months later they were sold. I was not quite sure what I wanted to do. I did not have the pressure of all the "kids" in college because they had all graduated but I certainly wanted to continue working. I heard through a grapevine of nurse friends that there was a part-time clinical instruction position at UNC Charlotte in Community Health Nursing open. I called to see if I qualified and possibly arrange an interview. I did qualify and I did arrange an interview. I was interviewed by Bill Cody, who was now PhD, Dr. Bill Cody! Here was my former friend and a person that I shared some nice NYC stories with, I felt right at home and the part-time job became a full-time job. I was thrilled to be out of the piranha life of certified home health agency and into a situation where there was intellectualization and collegiality. Several years later we discovered in conversation one evening that Bill had been hired for the community health lecturer when I turned it down. This is a story of "What goes around comes around" . . . and I am certainly glad that I came around.

MEREDITH FLOOD[12]

Step by Step

Each day as I travel across the campus of UNC Charlotte, I am reminded of how far our steps can take us though they may seem small at the moment. A particularly meaningful path of my route is the two sets of slate gray steps that must be climbed before approaching Colvard. There are 27 steps in all, which is the same age that I was upon starting the doctoral program at USC Columbia, an event that became a major turning point in my life. I first paid attention to the steps one day as I raced to Dr. Newman's psychiatric nursing class late (I was working third shift and had to attend class in the middle of my sleep time) and huffing and puffing. "I am 25 and I am out of breath going up these steps," but did not admit the shamefulness or gravity of what it meant.

Although it was not until the year after that the real changes started to occur. I recall that time of my life each day as I walk to Colvard. Now I don't even breathe hard. I am 60 pounds lighter and can run up the steps! I am not late. I am the one teaching the students now, hoping to reach them as a few special people at UNC Charlotte have reached out to me, touching my life personally and professionally. I think of how dramatically things have changed and I must credit much of my professional and academic growth to the people I am now privileged to call colleagues. I can honestly say I would not be where I am today if it weren't for Dr. Ann Newman and Dr. Jane Neese. They have provided encouragement and guidance, called me on the carpet when it was necessary, and believed in me when I did not. I believe I am in a special and unique position; I am very blessed to still be able to benefit from the expertise and wisdom of my former teachers, and am also in a role to reach out to my students the way that these special professors did for me. Going that extra mile for students does make a difference. Taking the time to know our students can have a lasting impression on them and can inspire those who may lack confidence and direction in their lives. The things we say and experiences we have with students may stay with them for years to come. This has been the case for me. I am inspired by those around me who have touched my life and motivated to do the same for my students.

MEREDITH TROUTMAN-JORDAN, UPDATE 2017[13]

It is now 14 years later, and how good it is to be reminded of why I am here at UNC Charlotte and what I strive to do. Now I am 44 years young, and still hiking steps and hills, though we are no longer in Colvard, but the beautiful College of Health and Human Services Building. And, I still walk this journey, step by step. There is a pretty path that can be walked from the Union Deck to our building, with budding flowers, young trees, and sunshine spilling down on many days. Colvard Building seems far away and foreign now. However, there is a great sense of belongingness and pride in being part of this family.

Many of our School of Nursing faculty have relocated or retired. I am now one of the most senior faculty here, in terms of the length of my time at UNC Charlotte. I am pleased to call Dr. David Langford (my former Community Health teacher!) and Mrs. Cynthia Toth (fellow "old faculty") colleagues. I also take any opportunity that exists to welcome new faculty, as I was so warmly welcomed when the path I traveled led me to UNC Charlotte. The start of this journey in 2003 was exciting and fun, and the trip continues to be challenging, yet exciting and very rewarding. Now I get to "pass on" the wisdom and kindness extended to me (by Dr. Newman, Dr. Neese, and Dr. Langford). I strive to do this through leadership roles, such as Sigma Theta Tau president and Systems MSN coordinator. I love my work and the people with whom I work.

There have been some dark valleys at points in my journey thus far, but there have been far more sunny hilltops. These are the parts that make the entire excursion so exciting and rewarding. I am now (re)married to a wonderful Christian man who I love more than I could ever imagine. I have a partner on my journey who encourages and supports me. Being in good health and having supportive family, loved ones, and professional colleagues makes a world of difference. I am encouraged and inspired to "pass on" the wisdom I have gained and the kindness and mentoring that others have provided me. It is critical that we, as nurses, do this, whether we are mentoring new staff nurses, fledgling nursing students, aspiring graduate nurses, or colleagues at any stage in their career. Mentoring and encouraging such individuals is a primary goal (and purpose, I have come to learn), of mine. I remain inspired by those around me who have touched my life and motivated to do the same for my students. I am "home," and yet the journey continues, step by step.

LIENNE EDWARDS[14]

My Story

My story goes back to the days when I was a new member of the nursing faculty. I remember the time fondly because of the teamwork, the peer support, and the collegiality that we had then. It seems pertinent to share it now because of our curriculum revision and the beginning of the new course.

The College of Nursing was implementing a new integrated curriculum (yes, we did say integrated curriculum!!) with Roy Adaptation Model as the framework. Each of four semesters of the junior and senior year had four courses, Adaptive Process, Nursing Process, Communication, and Roles. There was a team of us teaching each course, I especially remember Communications because I felt we really did good teamwork to teach this course. There were four of us faculty and we each had ¼ of the students in a seminar-type class (we admitted 120 students then). Each of us was responsible for preparing the content for a certain number of class topics. These materials were ready in advance and distributed to the other three faculty. We all met each week before class to review the materials and discuss teaching strategies for the topic. The meeting time was really beneficial; it was an on-going way of being consistent among the four groups and to have peer support for problems/issues that surfaced in one or more of the groups.

Not only did we have teamwork within courses, but we had it between courses as well. We regularly scheduled meetings of faculty teaching junior courses and of faculty teaching senior courses, I really felt the peer support from these groups. These experiences certainly did provide, as Bill said in his note to us, "identification, bonding, and good will" among us. When I think of these times and those people, I always remember it fondly.

DIANE DANIELS

A Good Beginning[15]

We talk a lot about caring in nursing. We implement "caring" into our curriculum. We "care" for our patients. However, there are times that we forget to apply these caring principles to our relationships with our colleagues. This was not the case when I began teaching at UNC Charlotte and is not the case now.

I began working as a TA and part-time clinical instructor at UNC Charlotte while finishing my master's degree. After completion of my degree, I was offered a lecturer position in the Adult Health Department. I left a small and very tight-knit group of colleagues with whom I had been teaching with for three years at a community college to begin my career at the university. I felt like a little bitty fish in a great big pond.

A month or so before the academic year began, I received a note from Gloria Hagopian. It was a simple message that had a tremendous impact. It basically stated, "So glad to hear you got the job. . . . I'm really looking forward to working with you. . . . If you need anything, just let me know." I immediately felt welcomed.

One of my greatest concerns about working at UNC Charlotte was that I had recently been a student in classes with the very same professors who would soon be my colleagues. Mary Curran and Gloria could not have made my transition to the role of colleague any smoother. From day one, they both reminded me that I also possessed a lot of knowledge and that they were there to offer their assistance. Beginning my career at UNC Charlotte with caring colleagues boosted my confidence level when I needed it most.

JACKIE DIENEMANN[16]

Candy

When applying, I was told the group of faculty had "strong personalities" and I would find working with them like "herding cats." So I was a little concerned as I went to meet these people. What did I find? A group that liked candy!

At the first department meeting in September I brought a bag of candy that everyone passed around as we went through the agenda. All went well. Afterward, Marilyn Smith came up and said she had actually enjoyed the meeting and its quick pace. Meanwhile, I had been meeting with faculty one by one in my office and found as we talked several took a mint out of the jar that the dean had given me as a welcome gift. I learned that Diane Daniels was enrolled in a doctoral program and taking two courses that semester. Sue Hartman and I shared being "temporary employees" and with uncertainty that comes with that—always good to have someone to commiserate with! I began to learn about who taught what, how the BSN program had Level 2 and Level 3, the Nurse Anesthesia program, the MSN/MHA and the Blended Role program, or rather the Advanced Practice Registered Nursing in Adult Chronic Care, or rather the APN/CNS Blended Role program. Boy, for a medical surgical focused group they sure were wordy in naming their master's programs. Over the next few months I learned the history of how the program evolved over the years.

By October, I brought a bag of candy again and we passed it around, and again we got a lot done in an hour. Mary Curran came up afterward and told me she liked that I was direct and followed the agenda. Linda Moore was working hard on the reaccreditation of the CRNA program; she would come by for a candy pick-me-up. I made a mistake when talking to Jim Steele about an issue without candy that took us a few months to clear up. Won't do that again.

As I got to know the faculty in the department I was impressed with many individual's expertise, scholarship, and teaching. Our department had the only faculty practice contract. This led to discussions in the department meeting about faculty practice. People in the department were proud of our accomplishments.

In November, I brought food, but not candy. It was passed around but not consumed like the candy, the meeting went slower. I had learned by lesson . . . this group liked candy! Despite the lack of candy, Mary got a CID grant funded that could support improvement of the NP program.

In December, we decided to go out to lunch rather than have a department meeting. That went well. Yes, I did bring candy that we shared. In January I brought jelly beans . . . that went better than any meeting had. So, after the meeting I put them on the refrigerator with a spoon . . . everyone was so cordial! I had figured it out: this group of "strong personalities" was just a group with low blood sugar!

Throughout the spring, I brought candy to our meetings and kept it on my desk. Low and behold, Shirley got the Late Life Long Term Care Academy approved. Sonya decided to apply for a post doc. Peggy, Dee, and Suzanne decided to apply again for funding of the Witnessing Project despite ACS turning them down again. Linda Steele decided to move the focus of her work to obesity management. Marilyn agreed to be our first community placement coordinator—that really required candy! Sue Hartman and I got hired in permanent positions. Sabrina got the John Biggs fellowship. This summer we heard Jim is now certified as an ANP. I bet he ate candy as he studied.

The only time I failed to remember to include candy this spring was in interviewing candidates for secretary . . . two people we offered the job turned it down . . .

should have given them candy at the interview. In July, we really did hire the right secretary. One of the first things Jan did was put a dish of Werther's Originals on top of the microwave. When that didn't move quickly, she added Tootsie Rolls. This woman had us figured out before I returned at the end of July. She knows how to build morale and create sweet moments. With a Tootsie Roll in your cheek, working on that syllabus doesn't seem too bad after all.

When on vacation this summer I got some huckleberry taffy. I have my fingers crossed that it will work as well as jelly beans at our first meeting in September.

CHAPTER SEVEN

Into a New Century, Implications/Adjustments to a New Structure

Dean Karen Schmaling, 2004–2010

Ann Mabe Newman

Karen Schmaling, PhD, became the first non-nursing dean of UNC Charlotte's College of Health and Human Services (CHHS) in 2004. She was extremely well qualified. She had a background in psychology and was a researcher with prolific publications. She became the dean of the Department of Social Work, Department of Kinesiology, Department of Health Behavior and Administration, and the School of Nursing (SON).

Dr. Schmaling began her first annual report[1] with the College of Health and Human Services' Top 10 Highlights for the academic year 2004–05:

Approval, accreditation, and initiation of new programs:

- The PhD program in Health Services Research was approved by the UNC Board of Governors on May 13, 2005, and became the college's first doctoral program.
- The Master of Science degree in Exercise Physiology was approved for the Department of Kinesiology.
- The Master of Social Work program was accredited by the Council on Social Work Education.
- The college's Learning Community, made up of students from each discipline in the CHHS enrolled its first cohort of students.

Educational partnerships with the community:

- The School of Nursing developed a new partnership with Carolinas Medical Center (CMC) and the Carolinas College of Health Sciences

(CCHS). UNC Charlotte SON will provide RN-to-BSN degree completion on the CMC/CCHS campus primarily for CMC employees and graduates of CCHS. More than 300 individuals at CCHS/CMC have expressed an interest in the program.

- The college has 112 affiliation agreements with community partners that collaborate to support the educational program.

Supporting our students:

- Nearly $34,000 in college-based scholarships were awarded to students this year.
- Two scholarships were awarded for the first time, and a scholarship fund for MSW students was started.

Research:

- Research being conducted by faculty in the departments of Health Behavior and Administration and Kinesiology is supported by grants from the National Institutes of Health.

Service:

- Most faculty members provide professional services and leadership to local, regional, state, and national entities.

Development and external relationships:

- We held the college's first Recognition and Awards Ceremony to honor our donors, faculty, students, scholarship recipients, and graduates.

The widely heralded nursing clinic at the Salvation Army Shelter for Homeless Women and Children was removed as a priority for the CHHS goals because it did not meet its established goals for the third year in row. A new era was clearly taking shape. Data were used to make some painful decisions. A plan was developed to remove the SON administrative responsibility for the nursing clinic by June 30, 2005. While most faculty understood why this decision was made, they were sad to see the university let go of the clinic. The College of Nursing had received so much goodwill in the community for meeting the needs of homeless women and children. Added value cannot always pay for itself in dollars.

The college faculty surveys indicated a need for research support. Dr. Schmaling responded by providing biostatistical support; funds were made available for an external reviewer to evaluate grant proposals; an incentive plan for research was developed; funds were offered to faculty members who wished to present a paper or attend a workshop on specific research skills. This new mandate for research was overwhelming to many of the nursing faculty. While it is true that the faculty needed to be encouraged to up its game in publishing, most were still novice researchers and resented the pressure this placed on them.

The 2005–06 School of Nursing's annual report[2] highlighted the following major accomplishments:

- 100% pass rate of nurse practitioner students on national certification exam.
- 100% pass rate of nurse anesthesia MSN students on national certification exam.
- Reorganization of SON structure approved through faculty governance and the UNC Board of Trustees effective July 1, 2006.
- Partnership with CMC and CCHS comes to fruition with the first RN/ BSN students admitted to the CMC cohort in August 2005.
- Development and approval of a faculty practice plan for the School of Nursing.
- Implementation of revised BSN and RN-BSN curricula.
- The School of Nursing Faculty Organization developed and approved a more-inclusive BSN admission policy for the fall of 2007.

While the report focused on what faculty did well and sounded quite positive, the executive summary was not as optimistic about reaching research funding goals.

Executive Summary of Annual Progress in Achieving 2005–2010 Strategic Plan Goals, Dr. Schmaling[3]

1. Programmatic and curricular issues/tracks moved forward during 2005–06 with new initiatives such as the e-learning grant that funded development of the nurse educator track as an online curriculum, implementation of revised BSN and RN/BSN curricula, and partial approval of the MSN program revisions. A faculty practice plan was approved by the faculty for implementation in the fall of 2006. Reorganization of the SON was approved through the governance process and will be implemented in 2006–07. However, one of the primary goals of the school—increased research and programmatic funding—did not occur. Submissions, in dollars, were half of what they were the previous year

2. Major new action steps planned to achieve goals in the 2005–10 strategic plan: This section was left blank.

3. Quality Enhancement Plan (QEP): Develop a QEP for the coming academic year. The National Council Licensure Examination (NCLEX pass rate for the past two classes of UNC Charlotte graduates was significantly lower (73% and 77%) than the national average. Some steps were taken as a result of 2004 results, but following the 2005 results, a comprehensive action plan was developed. The school piloted an NCLEX Improvement Plan during 2005–06. The effectiveness of this plan will not be apparent until the school receives the 2006 graduates' NCLEX pass rates:

- Implementation of case studies using a multi-specialty faculty team in all senior-level courses.
- Offer workshop on student clinical evaluation (August 2006; pilot was in May 2006).
- Devote half of senior leadership course to NCLEX review (by faculty and an outside NCLEX review consultant.
- Require that students receiving a lower than acceptable score on the nationally normed exit exam retake the exam with required advising with director, NCLEX improvement team, and/or advisor if scores were within a certain range.
- Establish benchmarks that denote an "at-risk" student (low exit exam scores, minority student)

Nursing faculty used their assessment skills to solve the problem of low NCLEX pass rates. We are so good at that. As a faculty member during this period of time, I am proud to report that the plan worked. In 2006, the school boasted a 98% NCLEX pass rate.

Since the change in structure, from a departmentalized College of Nursing to a School of Nursing within the UNC Charlotte College of Health and Human Services, changes were clearly necessary. Our growth and development was sometimes painful.

The 2006–07 year began under new administration for the School of Nursing with Dr. Lucille Travis, RN, PhD, joining the school as associate dean/director.

Dr. Travis brought warmth and enthusiasm to the SON. At our fall retreat, she presented us each with a big chocolate bar, labeled "A Successful School of Nursing." And the ingredients listed the names of each faculty member. We were off to another good start, continuing on our path of growth and development. The list of accomplishments for the year was amazing:

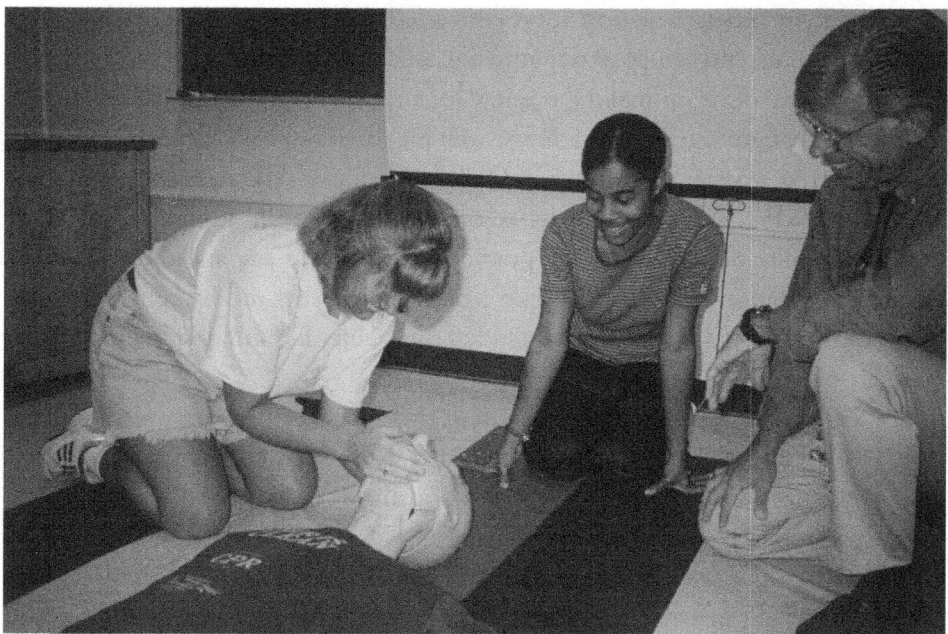

Nursing student learning how to perform CPR.

- Pass rate on NCLEX was 97%
- External grant proposals submitted were valued at $5.7 million
- Approved to offer MSN educator online
- Doubled admission of RN-to-BSN student in online program
- Received CCNE accreditation continuation for five years
- Dr. Jackie Dienemann, faculty member in the SON, appointed to Lake Norman Regional Medical Center Board of Trustees
- Stephanie Ramsey, RN/BSN student, named 2006 Great 100 Nursing Award Recipient
- Erika Jermaine Waters, BSN student, named 2006 Great 100 Nursing Scholarship Recipient
- Tracy Johnson and Dawn Swiderski, RN/BSN students, received AACN scholarships

With implementation of the new organizational structure, new administrative personnel, and a comprehensive review of programmatic offerings, goals were realigned to match the new initiatives and increased emphasis on scholarly productivity:

- Continue to monitor NCLEX pass rate. Maintain NCLEX pass rate at or above national benchmark
- Re-energize research

A three-year postgraduation survey revealed that 97% of BSN graduates reported being currently employed in nursing. All felt adequately or well prepared to apply an ethical decision-making framework and to provide culturally competent care. More than 90% felt adequately or well prepared to provide competent nursing care, act as a patient advocate, and delegate nursing responsibilities to others. Twenty-one MSN alumni responded to the survey, representing all three majors in the graduate program: 11 were nurse practitioners; 6 were nurse anesthetists; 4 were systems/population focused. Multiple written comments regarding the strength of the nursing program highly commended the faculty in both undergraduate and graduate programs.

Dr. Travis established a weekly newsletter to support transparent communication with faculty and staff and acknowledge faculty successes. Under the leadership of the new director, a positive "can do" attitude emerged, which resulted in increased productivity in all areas.

As 2007–08 highlights of the year, Dr. Lucille Travis outlined the following accomplishments in what she described as a very positive year for faculty and students:

Curricular/Enrollment Accomplishments: There was an increased admission to pre-licensure program of 10 students each semester of 2007–08. The RN-to-BSN online program doubled for a second year. Articulation agreements were completed with Gaston College, Stanley Community College, and Carolinas College of Health Sciences. The SON received approval from university administration to offer the Nurse Administrator program online through Distance Education.

Scholarly Accomplishments: Faculty submitted 32 proposals: 18 were research focused, 11 were programmatic, and 3 were student educational proposals. They sought a total of $6.6 million, representing a 14% increase from 2006–07. Faculty members published 16 articles, 4 books/chapters, and 16 articles were in press at the time of the annual report. Faculty also presented 19 research papers and posters and 13 other types of presentations.

Service/Community Accomplishments: In honor of the 40th anniversary of the first graduating class of the College of Nursing, a Distinguished Community Lectureship was offered to the Charlotte nursing community. Nearly 200 people attended. Our amazing undergraduate students contributed 76,140 hours to healthcare agencies via clinical service/learning. This fact is noteworthy in and of itself, but most especially because it represents the time investment of faculty in clinical supervision of students. In addition, graduate students contributed 28,740 hours to healthcare agencies via clinical/service learning.

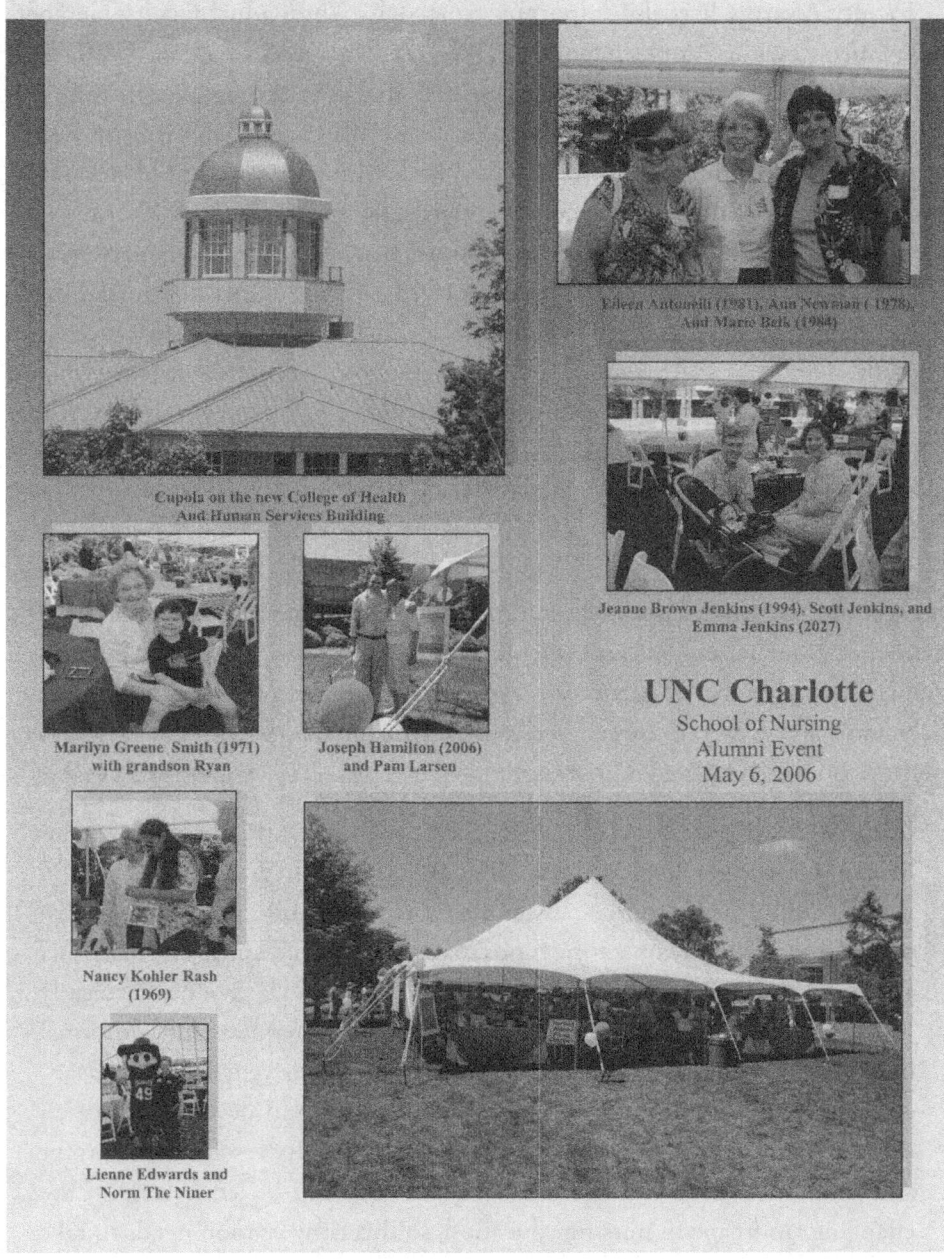

Fortieth anniversary Alumni Event program.

Faculty Awards: It is also important to recognize individual faculty members for some of their accomplishments. Dr. Maren Coffman and Dr. Peggy Wilmoth each received a prestigious American Nurses Foundation research grant. Wilmoth was selected as a Fellow in the American Academy of Nursing. Dr. Lienne Edwards was elected as chair of the North Carolina Nurses Association (NCNA) Commission on Education. Dr. Judy Cornelius received a federal subcontract. Dr. Meredith Flood received the Rising Investigator Award from Southern Nursing Research Society (SNRS). Dr. Ann Newman and Ms. Mary Smith received Nurse Educator Certification from NLN. Dr. Edwards and Dr. Tama Morris each received a Nursing Workforce HRSA grant. Dr. David Langford and Dr. Newman received an AHEC grant for the Nurse Educator Certificate program. Dr. Linda Moore was elected to the National Multiple Sclerosis Certification Board. Dr. Travis was elected secretary of the NC Council of Deans and Directors of Nursing and was chair of the AHEC regional Deans of Nursing Programs and Directors of Nursing Service.

According to the reports of the dean and the associate dean/director of the School of Nursing separate reports, Dr. Schmaling felt the college was doing well and Dr. Travis felt this was a successful year in the SON. However, friction between Schmaling and Travis continued to escalate. Dr. Schmaling wrote in her assessment of the School of Nursing for 2007–08:

> In 2008–09, the SON must be managed in such a way that promotes stabilization in order to facilitate its future development. In 2007–08, the SON received additional resources, including three new faculty positions and disproportionately more operating funds than other college units. The loss of six faculty to resignations and retirements in 2007–08 and lack of hires (in early June, 13 faculty positions were vacant) suggests that requests for additional lines in 2008–09 will be difficult to justify. The extensive number of vacancies jeopardizes our ability to offer the curriculum and develop a research enterprise. The curriculum must be aligned with faculty resources to current and future needs. I am concerned that the SON will be left behind in the changing landscape in nursing education, so this conversation needs to take place in 2008–09.[4]

In the summer of 2008, Dr. Travis resigned as associate dean/director of nursing and returned to faculty teaching.

Faculty were beginning to make great strides in writing grants and doing research, but were still feeling as if they could not keep up with expectations. There were many faculty vacancies, decreased resources to recruit new faculty, increased

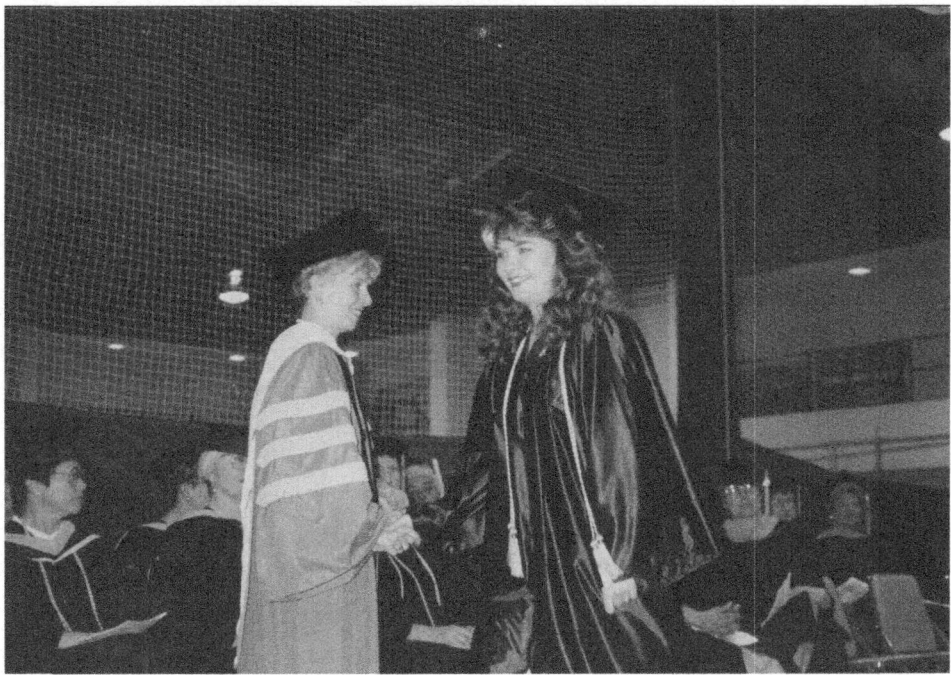

Dr. Barbara Carper, interim dean at graduation.

workloads, and the loss of yet another director of the SON. All of these things accumulated to decrease morale.

In 2008–09, Jane Neese, RN, PhD, associate dean of the College of Nursing and Health Profession, assumed the position of interim director of the School of Nursing. Once again, nursing faculty rose to the occasion. It was time to take responsibility for the future of our school and climb to the next level of development. Based on feedback received in 2007–08, throughout 2008–09 two committees of faculty and administrators reworked contentious sections of the Faculty Retention Tenure Promotion (ARTP) criteria in the faculty handbook.

CHAPTER EIGHT

Access and Partnerships

Pamala D. Larsen, PhD, RN, 2002–2006

On July 1, 2002, the College of Health and Human Services (CHHS) became the newest college at UNC Charlotte, replacing the former College of Nursing and Health Professions (CONHP). Within the college, the School of Nursing (SON) was formed as a semi-autonomous unit. The SON was the first school within a college at UNC Charlotte. Although plans for the new college and school had been in the making for some time, the UNC Charlotte Board of Trustees made it official in 2002.

The first two years of the new organizational structure was a time of learning who we were. Faculty governance for the new school was in place. However, there were still questions about how the school would function. Since the SON was the first school, there were no others on campus that could provide guidance. Would the SON operate or function differently from a college? How was the role of the SON different from the former College of Nursing and Health Professions? And perhaps more important, how would the SON act as a semi-autonomous unit? There were no magic answers to these questions. Thankfully, the Commission on Collegiate Nursing Education (CCNE) accreditation site visit was completed (re-accredited for 10 years in 2001), so the focus could be on moving forward and answering those questions.

The SON Advisory Board met for the first time in the fall of 2003. The board consisted of nursing leaders in acute care and community health and past alumni of UNC Charlotte. These leaders provided input on graduates' performances, current and future programs, and addressing the needs of the community. The board's guidance was critical at this stage in the SON's development.

In the first four years, access and partnerships best describe the work of the School of Nursing. During this time, the North Carolina Center for Nursing was pushing hard for baccalaureate-prepared nurses. In the early 2000s, the school had a small RN-BSN program. The majority of the courses were taught face-to-face on campus. Efforts were made to have one specific day of the week that courses would be taught, thus decreasing the number of days that students had to be on campus. These courses were supplemented with some online courses. Always a campus leader in distance education, the SON moved to expand its online offerings to provide better access for RN-BSN students. By 2003, in addition to the RN-BSN program on campus, an online RN-BSN program was offered. The early days of the online program had some ups and downs. Students were new to this kind of learning and often found it difficult. Additionally, there were issues with ownership of the online courses. It wasn't unusual for faculty members to leave the university and take their courses with them. Over the years, clearer guidelines were established with assistance from the university attorney. Also, in prior years, the rule was that if a student had taken certain prerequisite courses, anatomy and physiology for example, more than 10 years earlier, they had to retake the courses. This was not a popular part of the program among RNs who had completed their education more than 10 years ago, and removing this requirement boosted enrollment in the RN-BSN program.

In 2004–05, the SON received funding from UNC Charlotte's Office of the President and an e-learning initiative on campus to partner with the School of Nursing at UNC Wilmington to develop a RN-BSN curriculum that could be shared. So, if one school was not offering a particular online course that semester, it would be available to students at the other school. The idea was to provide more options for RN-BSN students.

In 2005, Carolinas College of Health Sciences (CCHS) and Carolinas Medical Center (CMC) partnered to offer RN-BSN courses and some prerequisites on their campuses in Charlotte. That year, RN students from CMC and second-year students at CCHS were able to take courses on the CMC campus. The addition of the CMC site gave students a third option for RN-BSN education.

In the fall of 2005, the first students were admitted to the PhD program in Health Services Research in the College of Health and Human Services (CHHS). The program was a culmination of several years of effort between the Department of Social Work, Department of Health Behavior and Administration, and the School of Nursing, since they were now housed together in the College of Health and Human Services.

The graduate programs at UNC Charlotte SON continued to grow. The Nurse Anesthesia program, offered through a partnership with the CMC, was a strong program with 100% of students passing the national exam each year. Smaller programs, such as the community health and psychiatric clinical nurse specialist

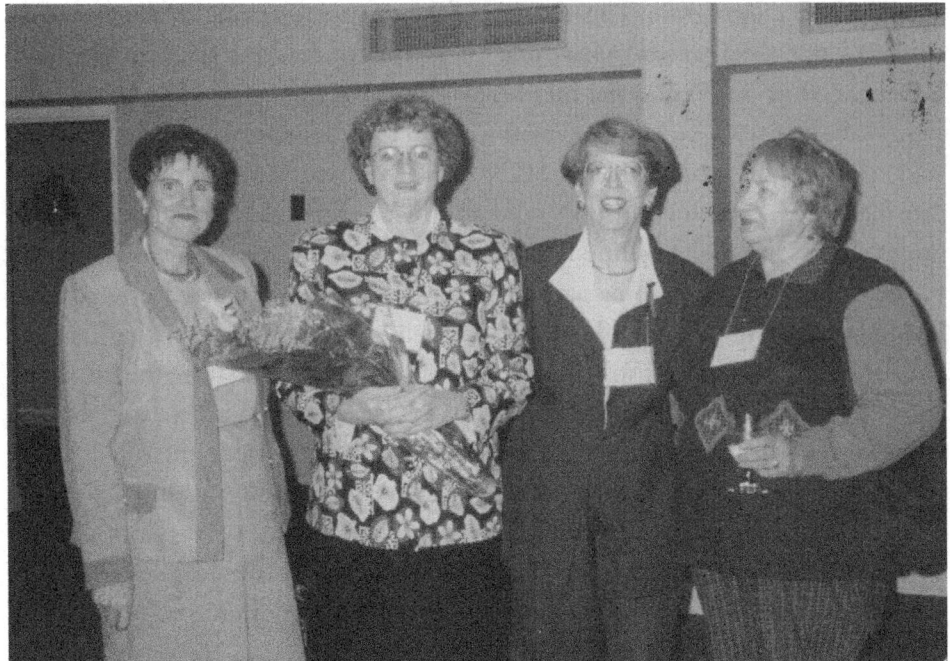

Jerre Jones, RN, PMH, CNS; Gerry Roberts, RN, MSN, president of NCNA;
Ann Mabe Newman, RN, PhD, all UNC Charlotte CON graduates with Dr. Sally
Nicholson, RN, PhD, UNC Charlotte faculty at NCNA Convention.

tracks, were not offered every year, but every other year. In 2006, the adult nurse
practitioner/clinical nurse specialty (ANP/CNS) track was phased out in favor of
the family nurse practitioner (FNP) program, a more popular program with students. In contrast, the combined master's in nursing/master's in nursing/master's in
Health Administration (MSN/MHA) track had a lower number of students than
expected, and preliminary planning began for a nurse administrator track instead
of the dual degree.

The nurse educator certificate program was the first step in the development of a
nurse educator track. Nursing faculty from community colleges had long asked for
courses that would supplement their knowledge and ability to teach. Many of those
faculty came from clinical practice and did not have a background in teaching. The
nurse educator certificate program was launched in the summer of 2003, and the
nurse educator track followed.

The BSN program had long been a stalwart in the community. Typically, 100
students were admitted each fall. Although there was talk of increasing the number of BSN students each year, the decreasing number of clinical sites prevented

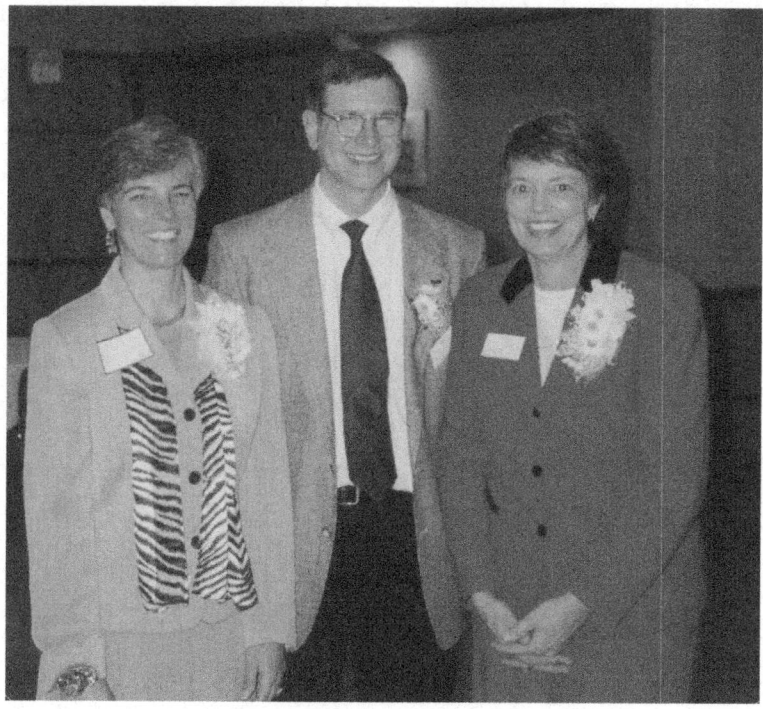

Dr. Larsen with first Colvard scholar.

any change in enrollment. An increasing number of schools of nursing, offering both baccalaureate and associate degrees, competed for the limited number of sites. UNC Charlotte SON students often had clinical courses during the evenings or on weekends.

A new BSN curriculum was developed and offered for the first time in the fall of 2005. One new feature of the program was the admission of 50 students each semester versus 100 once a year. This gave the students who had to repeat a course or drop out because of personal reasons an option to get back into the program the next semester instead of waiting until the next year.

Although UNC Charlotte SON was established in 2002, the school's infrastructure remained as it had when it was the College of Nursing. The two departments, Adult Health Nursing and Family and Community Nursing, shared both undergraduate and graduate programs. Each department had a chair that reported to the director of the SON. This arrangement became more cumbersome as the years passed, and it did not help unify faculty under the school structure. In the fall of 2006, a new infrastructure was implemented with one department for undergraduate studies and one for graduate studies. Each of these departments was led by a chair.

The first four years at the SON was an exciting time. In becoming a school, a new vision for the future developed. The robustness of being in a larger college spurred new partnerships with other departments and faculty. The school was moving forward.

CHAPTER NINE

UNC Charlotte's Golden Anniversary and Beyond

Dean Nancy Fey-Yensan, PhD, RD, College of Health
and Human Services, 2011–Present (2018)

Of the nursing profession, President Barack Obama once said, "America's nurses are the beating heart of our medical system." On that, I enthusiastically agree. Further, I would venture to say that at the University of North Carolina at Charlotte, our nursing program, one of the university's first programs, has been at the heart of what has grown to be a dynamic College of Health and Human Services. The evolution of nursing at the university has been a reflection of the profession's evolution. Nursing has propelled so many important aspects of modern-day medicine and health care—public health, physical therapy, and dietetics—just to name a few. Our nursing program has contributed much to strengthen the health disciplines represented in the college, while continuing to evolve in its own right, thriving as a driving force in research, and engaging in community service. For these reasons, nursing has become one of the most sought-after degree programs at UNC Charlotte.

The College of Health and Human Services, founded in 1996, already had an ambitious agenda when I arrived in the summer of 2011. I inherited a college that was well on its way to making its mark on Charlotte, the region, the state, and the country. Dr. Jane Neese, a tenured faculty member in the School of Nursing and acting associate dean for the college since the departure of Dean Karen Schmaling in 2010, had been named interim dean by Provost Joan Lorden. For more than a year, Dr. Neese dedicated herself to ensuring that the college stayed on track academically while continuing to pursue innovation and service. It is with much gratitude that I acknowledge Dr. Neese for her outstanding work on behalf of the college during this time between deans. She was, and remains, a strong leader and advocate for all of our academic programs, but has a special affinity for the School of Nursing. It was through her that I learned quickly of the school's prominence and promise. We rapidly hit our stride together, and now as the senior associate dean of the College of Health and Human Services, Dr. Neese remains tireless in her promotion of the school and her support of its faculty, staff, and students.

A Talented Faculty Educates Future Nurses

The talent needed to fuel a contemporary nursing program has changed considerably since the inception of our program more than 50 years ago. There are four types of faculty in the School of Nursing who make significant contributions every day to our three-part mission to teach, conduct research, and engage in community service. Our lecturers and clinical professors, who are largely responsible for the heavy lifting in our classrooms, teach in laboratories and in the hundreds of clinical settings our students rotate through as part of their training to become bachelor's-prepared nurses or to earn a master's or DNP degree. Our tenure-track professors, also essential teachers and mentors, split their time between educating students at all levels and conducting cutting-edge research. And, we could not do what we do, meeting such high standards, without the scores of amazing adjunct faculty who elect to teach didactic or clinical courses for us. Many of these practicing nurses are our own BSN, MSN, and DNP graduates. Importantly, they are on the front lines every day and bring a perspective that enriches our curriculum and prepares our students to "hit the ground running" after graduation. In order to keep current and maintain their credentials, our nursing faculty regularly engage in professional and clinical skills development and return to the classroom with fresh perspectives to add to their teaching. I believe that, in part, it is their commitment to their own development that results in graduates who are the most sought-after nurses in the region.

It is really important to acknowledge that in the College of Health and Human Services, more than 40% of our students are the first in their families to go to college, and that 75% of our students need financial support. Understanding the students' needs and the need for a diverse student body in order to produce a diverse and effective workforce, the School of Nursing has worked for the past 10 years to design and implement support programs funded by a variety of sources, most notably Health Resources and Services Administration (HRSA) (DHHS). An impressive $4.4 million in student support has been provided to our students who might otherwise have left the university not because of ability or academic performance, but because of financial need.

Whether our nursing students are taught by a lecturer, clinical professor, tenure-track professor, or an adjunct faculty member, they are being challenged and nur-

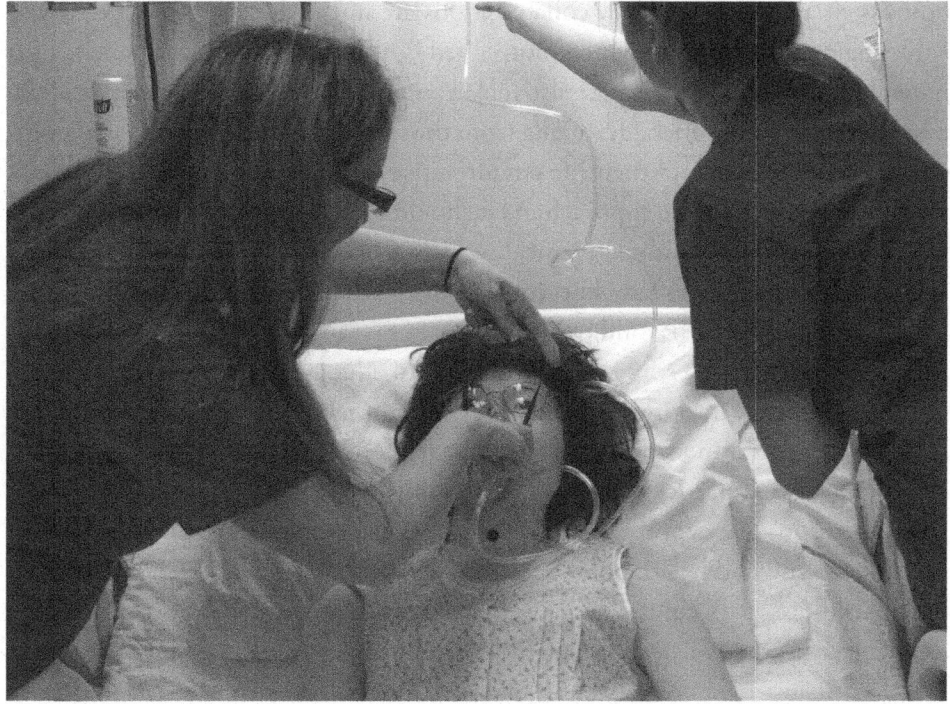

Student in simulation lab in the 2010s.

tured, principles that I know Miss Bonnie believed in and would approve of. In the almost seven years I have served as dean at UNC Charlotte College of Health and Human Services (CHHS) I have been immensely impressed with and appreciative of how student-centric our faculty are; they are attentive to environmental, economic, and social shifts that may require adjustments in pedagogy and approaches to mentoring. One telling outcome of the faculty's commitment to student success has been the climbing and remarkable pass rates on the National Council Licensure Examination (NCLEX). In the spring of 2017, it was 98%—a record for the school and a testament to the vision and energy of some of the very best teachers at the UNC Charlotte.

A Growing Capacity for Research and Discovery

In addition to their dedication to educational excellence at both the undergraduate and graduate levels, School of Nursing faculty are also committed to scholarly discovery and innovation. What is particularly impressive is the scope of their research and the potential impact of their results. Nurse scholars are keenly aware of how essential interdisciplinary collaborations are in the discovery process; it was a nursing foundation from which most allied health professions have hailed. This natural inclination to collaborate also makes sense in the context and analysis of the nursing care model, which, departing from the traditional medical model, considers the whole patient and their life circumstances when making decisions about a treatment or preventative approach. As it should be and has often happened in the history of nursing, traditional medical models are being adjusted and more often aligned with what nurses have known and practiced all along—effective outcomes for patients that go far beyond treating disease.

The trajectory of research in the School of Nursing over the past 10 years (2007–present) is tracking with the school's high marks in teaching. Our nurse scholars are experts in using a variety of research techniques such as clinical trials, community-based participatory research, health informatics, mobile technology, and simulation. They apply their deep knowledge and passion to bring us closer to solutions for myriad health issues related to poverty, health equity, homelessness, psychiatric disorders, and military service. This includes diabetes, HIV/AIDS, asthma, cardiovascular disease, maternal/infant/child health, and mental/behavioral health, just to name a few. Our talented nurse scholars are also tackling some of the most troubling social and health-related phenomenon of the day—early childhood trauma, interpersonal violence, and substance abuse—through their research and community engagement. I have also been struck by our faculty's commitment to bringing their deep knowledge directly back to the community as they dedicate hours to providing free or low-cost continuing education credits for practicing nurses working in our school systems, acute care settings, community clinics, long-term care, non-profit agencies, and veteran services.

Over a period of 10 years, the School of Nursing has received 80 research awards totaling about $9.4 million from federal and local governmental sources, private foundations, professional associations, nongovernment organizations, nonprofits, and business and industry. Importantly, the number of grant submissions when compared to grant awards indicates a success rate of more than 60% in the past two years, and almost 50% over the past decade. This is a true point of pride and a robust indicator of the potential for research at the School of Nursing.

An Essential Community Partner
in Improving Life Quality and Health

One of the major reasons I was so excited to come to Charlotte as the dean of the College of Health and Human Services was that I could see the tremendous potential for the college to have an increasingly powerful and positive impact on a variety of quality-of-life dimensions in Charlotte, the county, the region, and the state. Nurses are among the most natural community connectors. Our faculty demonstrate their ability in communities of need every day and bring this passion to their students as well. Very early in their education, all of our students, whether they are at the bachelor's, master's, or doctoral level, understand the absolute commitment of our faculty to community engagement and learn that this engagement must also be in their portfolios as practitioners. Without fail, if I am asked to find faculty to provide community presentations as subject matter experts or to represent the college at community fairs, outreach events, or our statewide UNC Charlotte Science Expo, our School of Nursing faculty and their students are the first to volunteer. In addition, our talented faculty provide hours of service sharing their expertise on nonprofit boards, volunteering in local clinics, and as medical providers through international medical mission trips during their spring breaks, the summer, and even holidays. They are a remarkable and generous faculty who set the bar for community service extremely high.

The Horizon Is Bright for the School of Nursing

Evolving from an enrollment of fewer than 10 students in the 1960s to being one of UNC Charlotte's first accredited programs in the 1970s, our nursing program continues to be a beacon of academic excellence. It is the oldest pillar of the College of Health and Human Services, and of that we are very proud. I consider the School of Nursing's capacity and mission as clearly embracing the two words in the college's name—"health" and "human." Increasing NCLEX pass rates, the employment statistics of our graduates, our growing research enterprise, our commitment to and success in increasing the diversity of our faculty and students, and our commitment to engage in the local and broader community are strong indicators that the School of Nursing has run a good race. But, as we all know, that's not the end of our story. We are only hitting our stride. There are so many more lives and systems to change and improve. The School of Nursing has enjoyed tremendous success in its first 50 years and is poised for continued success in the next 50 years.

CHAPTER TEN

Recognition, Successes, New Programs in Nursing

Dee M. Baldwin, PhD, RN, FAAN,
Associate Dean/Director, 2009–2017

It was my honor to serve the University of North Carolina at Charlotte as associate dean and director of the School of Nursing from 2009–17. During my eight-year tenure, we accomplished much to sustain the school's growth. Building on the work of previous administrations, the school generated several new academic programs and came up with the concept of "Niner Nurses," a recognition for alumni concept used to denote the ways in which the school prepared our students as leaders, experts, scholars, and partners to make a difference in the lives of the people we serve. The school also raised its profile nationwide with soaring licensure and certification rates, creation of the UNC Charlotte/WCU Dual Doctoral of Nursing Practice (DNP) program, and the achievement of a National League for Nursing (NLN) Center of Excellence designation for Creating Environments that Enhance Student Learning and Professional Development. Further, our partners, donors, advisory board members, and friends continued to work side by side with us to help preserve and protect our legacy, while our faculty and staff continue to produce top graduates and leaders in health care.

School of Nursing Highlights (2009–2017)

Academics and Enrollment

In 2009, enrollment saw more than 900 applicants competing for 100 available slots in the undergraduate nursing program. As a campus, UNC Charlotte had exceeded its growth projections in numbers of students as well as academic programs. Likewise, our pre-nursing student enrollment was growing, but the nursing major became one of the most highly sought-after majors on campus, so we were turning away many qualified students. To respond to the students' needs, in 2010 the school launched an aggressive enrollment management plan to decrease the overall numbers of pre-nursing students. The plan was a huge success as numbers of pre-nursing students dramatically decreased by 56%, dropping from 941 in the fall of 2010 to 419 in the fall of 2013. The school also worked with the college to add new undergraduate programs to provide pre-nursing students not admitted to the nursing program with additional options for attaining a health-related career.

Sustaining and Enhancing Academic Programs through Strong Community Partnerships

The school, well known in the Charlotte community for its strong academic programs and innovative learning environments, continued its instructional programming that focused on those successes that were responsive to the needs of the community and to society as a whole. For example, the school doubled its enrollment in the RN-to-BSN program by offering an early entry option to further enhance opportunities to associate degree nurses. The school partnered with three community colleges to launch this key initiative to increase access to baccalaureate nursing education for graduates of associate degree nursing (ADN) programs.

In addition to the early option entry, the school added a Centralina Regionally Increasing Baccalaureate Nurses (CRIBN) option, a seamless pathway from associate degree to the BSN degree via a collaborative partnership of baccalaureate and associate degree nursing programs. CRIBN admitted its first cohort of eight students to the RN-to-BSN program in May 2015. Centralina RIBN was one of eight North Carolina partnerships designed to increase the number of nurses with a baccalaureate degree. Our CRIBN partners were located at UNC Charlotte, Gaston College, Central Piedmont Community College, and Carolinas College of Health Sciences. The first cohort of ADN students graduated from UNC Charlotte's RN-to-BSN program in May 2016.

The School of Nursing reached a major milestone in 2013 with the establishment of the UNC Charlotte/Carolinas HealthCare System (HCS) Adult Gerontology Acute Care Nurse Practitioner (AGACNP) collaborative. This program, the only one of its kind in the Charlotte region, was added to the School of Nursing's MSN program to improve the health outcomes of patients experiencing episodes of acute care and as a clinical experience for students. The program assisted in delivering health care to an onslaught of patients at CHS due to implementation of the Affordable Care Act, while exposing student practitioners to leaders in a variety of health specialties: nurses, physicians, and experts in psychology, bioinformatics, simulation, and other fields. Graduates of the collaborative exited as master's-prepared nurse practitioners and experts in the care of acutely ill patients with complex problems. Certification rates within these programs soared during this period, ranging from 92% to 100% for both the Family Nurse Practitioner (FNP) and Adult Geriatric Acute Care Nurse Practitioner (AGACNP) options.

Another historic event that occurred in 2013 was the creation of the Doctor of Nursing Practice (DNP) program, a joint project of UNC Charlotte and Western Carolina University (WCU). The UNC Charlotte/WCU Dual DNP program was approved by the University of North Carolina System General Administration in February 2013, and became the 20th doctoral program offered on UNC Charlotte's campus and the first doctoral program offered in the School of Nursing. The DNP program admitted its first cohort in 2013, and the program at both institutions continues today to share a common curriculum, the same admission and progression policies, and degree requirements. The program also shares faculty, marketing, library, and other resources.

Other accomplishments during the 2009–17 period included the reaccreditation of all academic programs. In 2011, the Commission on Collegiate Nursing Education (CCNE) reaccredited the school's baccalaureate and master's programs for 10 years, noting no violations in standards of practice during its comprehensive review. This accomplishment, a major achievement for the school, validated our high standards as the purpose of national accreditation is to confirm program quality.

In 2014, the Nurse Anesthesia (NA) program was reaccredited for 10 years by the Commission on Accreditation (COA) for Nurse Anesthesia Education programs. The NA program, which received a positive review, enjoyed only commendations with no compliance violations. In 2016, our newly created UNC Charlotte/WCU Dual DNP program received initial CCNE accreditation for a five-year period, and the school served as the lead organization of this collaborative with the associate dean and director, Dr. Dee Baldwin, RN, named the first chief nurse administrator of the dual-degree program.

Student Success as Evident
through National Prominence and Rankings

As early as 2000, the school's strategic plan detailed an approach to reach national prominence through excellence in creative and innovative teaching/learning environments, those that encourage student success and produce exceptional graduates. Two major accomplishments speak to the school's progress in reaching its goal of national prominence. First, in 2015, the school's online graduate programs jumped in national rankings from 87 to 54 as noted and reported by *US News & World Reports.*[1] This jump occurred as a result of the strengthening of the infrastructure of the school by incorporating an admissions officer to solely address the skyrocketing number of applications to the various tracks in the MSN program, employing a records and admission specialist to attend to student application questions and flexible and new innovative curricula offered in the graduate programs (MSN and Dual DNP). These efforts offered quality programs and strengthened communications between faculty, new and continuing students, and staff.

Second, the school achieved designation as a National Center of Excellence by the National League for Nursing in the area of Creating Environments That Enhance Student Learning and Professional Development. This accomplishment, based on the school's ability to present its model of teaching/learning through the conceptualization and specification of a values-based education and evidence-based practice curriculum, was noted by the organization as one that focuses on student success and excellence.

Additionally, the UNC Charlotte/WCU Dual DNP degree program advanced the national prominence of the school through vigorous efforts related to marketing and recruitment of students. During this period, the faculty continued to raise the school's profile with their appointments and selections to national organizations, including the American Academy of Nursing, Society of Pediatric Nursing, American Heart Association (AHA), and International Nurses Society on Addictions, to name a few.

Research, Scholarship, and Funding

School of Nursing faculty continued to develop active programs of research and state-of-the-art educational activities related to vulnerable populations during the 2009–17 period. The school focused its energy on becoming a model for research on vulnerable populations such as aging, health disparities, and chronic illnesses. UNC Charlotte's goal to be recognized as North Carolina's urban university inspired the faculty to expand their research even more to include community engagement activities and work with underserved and diverse groups. For example, faculty researching issues associated with child maltreatment worked with the Mecklenburg County Health Department School Health Nurses program to address child abuse in the Charlotte community and beyond. The school made a commitment to connect with other disciplines and engage community partners to improving the health of the communities we served. The school also saw steady and continuous research funding from national agencies including the National Institutes of Health, American Nurses Foundation, U.S. Department of Health and Human Services, the U.S. Department of Defense, SAMHSA, and various other funding sources. We continued to support the faculty by providing doctoral and graduate students as research assistants, paying consultants to review and edit publications and proposals, funding intramural pilot projects (such as the School of Nursing Director's Research and Scholarship fund), and providing funds for travel to present at state, national, and international conferences.

In 2009, the school received funds for two endowed chairs, the Carol Grotnes Belk Endowed Chair and the Dean W. Colvard Distinguished Professorship. Both awards were designated for junior faculty members and were intended to strengthen their teaching and research programs. In 2013, the dean of the College of Health and Human Services Nancy Fey-Yensan expanded the scope of the Dean W. Colvard Distinguished Professorship and moved it from the school to the college to encourage scholarly contributions from the interdisciplinary community to research, teaching, and mentoring.

During my tenure, the school also received two large Health Resources and Services Administration (HRSA) Nursing Workforce Diversity grants to provide opportunities to undergraduate students seeking BSN degrees. In 2014, a grant entitled "Crossing Borders: Making Connections," under the leadership of the associate director of the Undergraduate Division, was given almost $1 million for a three-year period. The grant provided for 10 additional students from economic and/or educational disadvantaged backgrounds to be admitted to the university each academic year of the funding period. The program also included curriculum enhancement events related to diversity and provided faculty development activities on diversity-related topics.

The second grant, the HRSA Nursing Workforce Diversity Grant, was funded in 2012–16 in the amount of $2.3 million. This grant, also overseen by the undergraduate associate director, provided scholarships to students from disadvantaged backgrounds so they could complete the undergraduate nursing program. This grant also provided academic success strategies, expanded multicultural experiences, and implemented a holistic review process in an effort to increase and promote a more diverse workforce.

The William Randolph Hearst Foundation (WRHF) continued to support graduate education through the WRHF Scholars program. The long-term goal of this program was to prepare a more diverse advanced practice and graduate nursing workforce, one that will provide culturally competent nursing care. Our application in the amount of $100,000, renewed twice during the 2009–17 period, provided much-needed financial support. In addition, the school submitted competitive applications annually to the Health Resources and Services Administration (HRSA) Traineeship Grant program for the Nurse Anesthesia program and was extremely

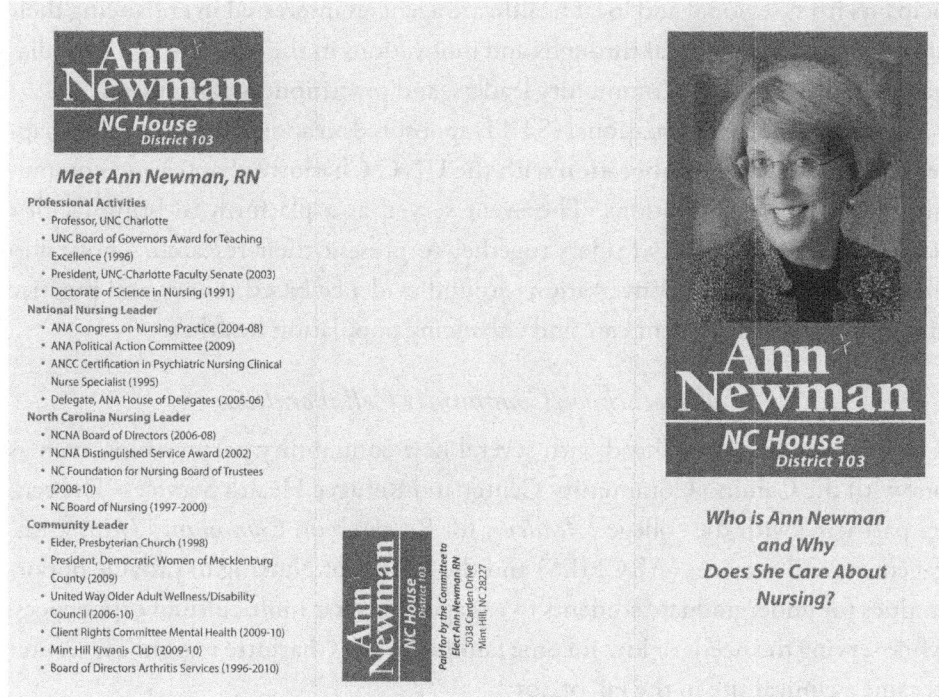

Meet Ann Newman, RN

Professional Activities
- Professor, UNC Charlotte
- UNC Board of Governors Award for Teaching Excellence (1996)
- President, UNC-Charlotte Faculty Senate (2003)
- Doctorate of Science in Nursing (1991)

National Nursing Leader
- ANA Congress on Nursing Practice (2004-08)
- ANA Political Action Committee (2009)
- ANCC Certification in Psychiatric Nursing Clinical Nurse Specialist (1995)
- Delegate, ANA House of Delegates (2005-06)

North Carolina Nursing Leader
- NCNA Board of Directors (2006-08)
- NCNA Distinguished Service Award (2002)
- NC Foundation for Nursing Board of Trustees (2008-10)
- NC Board of Nursing (1997-2000)

Community Leader
- Elder, Presbyterian Church (1998)
- President, Democratic Women of Mecklenburg County (2009)
- United Way Older Adult Wellness/Disability Council (2006-10)
- Client Rights Committee Mental Health (2009-10)
- Mint Hill Kiwanis Club (2009-10)
- Board of Directors Arthritis Services (1996-2010)

Ann Newman
NC House
District 103

Paid for by the Committee to Elect Ann Newman RN
5038 Carden Drive
Mint Hill, NC 28227

Who is Ann Newman and Why Does She Care About Nursing?

Ann Newman first advanced practice RN to run for NC legislature.

successful in receiving financial support each year for students completing their degrees.

Community Engagement

Community engagement remained a strategic goal and priority of the school, college, and university. The school viewed the term broadly to include: (1) ongoing community partnerships to strengthen our curricula and hosting mutually beneficial programming to address urgent healthcare and professional issues, (2) collaborating with the college to promote health in the community, (3) serving on community and professional boards, and (4) partnering with students and alumni. These goals are outlined in more detail below.

Ongoing Mutually Beneficial Community Programs

During the 2009–17 period, the school engaged in a number of community programs. For several years, the school co-hosted with Charlotte AHEC an annual diabetes conference. This program was attended annually by more than 200 participants from regional and local healthcare agencies interested in enhancing their knowledge on recent breakthroughs and innovations in the care of those with diabetes. Faculty, students, community leaders, and practitioners participated.

Sigma Theta Tau International (STTI) sponsored an annual Gamma Iota Chapter Research Day in collaboration with the UNC Charlotte chapter and community healthcare organizations. The event served as a platform to bring faculty, students, and community leaders together to present their research/scholarship findings and engage in conversations around evidence-based theory and practice aimed at improving patient care and enhancing population health.

College/School/Community Collaborations

The school also forged ahead with several new community partnerships, such as one with the Camino Community Center and Refugee Health Services. The center partnered with the college's *Academy* for Research on *Community Health,* Engagement and Services (ARCHES) and the School of Nursing to provide opportunities for undergraduate students to engage in diverse multicultural experiences, while serving the needs of low-income families in the Charlotte region. The center became a clinical site in the fall of 2017.

In 2016, the school joined forces with the Mecklenburg County Health Department to include Refugee Health Services as an integral part of the students' community health rotation. According to North Carolina population projections, more than 700 individuals from around the world move to Charlotte each year as refugees. This school-county partnership provides a service to the citizens of North Carolina by assisting with the resettlement process and providing health education to newly arrived families while simultaneously enhancing the training of our students to work with diverse populations.

Engagement through Service on Community Boards

School of Nursing faculty continued to embrace the mission of improving population health by being actively involved in community organizations and serving on a number of boards during the 2009–17 period. Our faculty and students, connecting with healthcare providers, professional organizations, schools, businesses, and patient groups, continued to work with leaders in the communities and healthcare institutions to address the healthcare needs of the Charlotte Mecklenburg County area and beyond. These needs focused on enhancing health, education, and the environment, with the goal of improving health outcomes and quality of life for members of the community. Our relationship with community stakeholders facilitated a mutually beneficial exchange of knowledge and resources in a context of partnership and reciprocity. Examples of engagement activities by school faculty and staff included: (1) leadership roles on health-related community boards, (2) community education about HIV, diabetes, obesity, and physical activity, (3) disaster preparedness education, (4) health screenings and education fairs for targeted populations, and (5) faculty practices in community settings.

Students, Graduates, and Alumni Success Stories That Affect Communities

Our students, graduates, and alumni have had much success and a real impact in the communities they serve. In 2014, one of our senior nursing students was one of 109 students chosen out of more than 800 across the country for a summer externship at the Mayo Clinic in Minnesota, consistently ranked as one of the top five hospitals in the United States. The student gained clinical experience, networked with a diverse group of peers, and learned from some of the best minds in health care.

Another success story was that of Kailey Filter, a BSN 2015 graduate. In 2014, she served as a cadet training assistant for ROTC students attending field training at Maxwell Air Force Base in Alabama and was named Training Assistant of the Year in 2016. At UNC Charlotte, she was the university's top ROTC student, known as the Cadet Wing Commander, responsible for leading 80 cadets through military training. The year she graduated, 2015, she was selected as the #1 Air Force ROTC cadet in the southeast region of the United States out of 3,494 cadets, and #3 nationwide out of 10,883 cadets. She was commissioned by the U.S. Air Force as a second lieutenant upon graduation.

In 2012, UNC Charlotte's Association of Nursing Students (ANS) was recognized by the city of Charlotte's Philanthropy Foundation for spearheading the creation of the Ashley Lutz Memorial Scholarship. This scholarship in the amount of $25,000, an Endowed Scholarship in memory of a deceased classmate, was created in collaboration with the CHHS development office, the Gamma Iota Chapter of Sigma Theta Tau, and the Lutz family, and was recognized as the only one of its kind to be created by students at UNC Charlotte. ANS also initiated and participated in a number of community events during this period, including fundraising for the Ronald McDonald House, Hospitality House, and volunteering for the Carolina Blood Bank blood drive, Susan G. Komen Race for the Cure, Second Harvest Food Bank, and Walk to End Alzheimer's Disease. Our students also participated in multiple on-campus activities, including an ANS mentor-mentee program, ANS clothing drive, and Jamil Niner food pantry.

While strengthening their clinical skills and enhancing their research capabilities, our graduate students remained a priority. Professional development and community engagement continued as a major focus of the curriculum during the 2009–17 period. Our MSN students enjoyed much success in their research projects, spurred by their coursework in research synthesis. For example, in 2015, the CRNA students took first and third place in poster presentations at a statewide student competition at the annual Student Nurse Anesthesia Conference. Also, that year MSN students presented their research projects at the Gamma Iota Sigma Theta Tau Research Day, taking first-, second-, and third-place awards, and a people's choice poster award. Our DNP students, mentored by our faculty, successfully presented and defended their final scholarly projects in 2015 and presented them at the Gamma Iota Annual Research Day.

The School of Nursing reenergized its School of Nursing Alumni Chapter (SONAC) with help from the college's Development Office and University Office of Alumni Affairs in 2011. In 2012, the university recognized SONAC as the first academic alumni chapter on UNC Charlotte's campus. In addition, the SONAC, partnering with the community, university, and school, began sponsoring an annual Distinguished Nursing Alumni Lectureship, which brought together leading professionals in a multidisciplinary setting to network and discuss cutting-edge healthcare issues. At each annual conference, a Distinguished Alumni Award is presented to a UNC Charlotte nursing alumnus for outstanding service to the School of Nursing, exceptional achievement, or state/national/international leadership. Five outstanding alumni have received this award since 2011.

In closure, during my tenure from 2009–17, the school had many accomplishments, but I am most proud of the growth of the school's academic programs and collaborations with local, regional, and national partners. I am equally proud of the school's continuous focus on diversity. When I arrived at UNC Charlotte, the faculty was 5% nonwhite. Upon my exit, minorities made up 19.4% of the faculty. While this is a modest increase, I believe recruitment and retention of a diverse faculty and student body is essential if the school is to fulfill its mission to prepare nursing professionals to meet the healthcare needs of a diverse society. Finally, I am so proud of the accomplishments of our students. They enter as novices and exit as experts, leaders, partners, and scholars. I credit our outstanding, talented, and dedicated School of Nursing faculty, staff, and alumni. I remain honored and privileged to have served this great school.

Student Memories, 2000s

ALY BELL, RN, BSN, CLASS OF 2011[2]

The UNC Charlotte nursing program was rigorous and demanding, much like my other full-time job of being a single mom to a two year old! It was also fulfilling, rewarding, awe-inspiring, terrifying, and amazing—also much like being a single mom! My son inspired me through all of the challenges and hurdles of nursing school to constantly strive to be a better student and a better person.

The year 2011 was marked by several events that stand out clearly in my memory. It was a year of celebration and sadness. The Navy Seals took down Osama bin Laden. Steve Jobs passed away. Prince William married Kate Middleton. Kim Jong-il passed on and left Kim Jong-un in power. Congresswoman Gabrielle Gifford was injured in a horrific shooting. The spacecraft Juno launched. It was a time of turmoil, hope, and change in the Middle East during the Arab Spring movement.

It was an exciting time to be a nursing student—we had amazing facilities at UNC Charlotte School of Nursing that allowed us to take part in simulation labs and to practice our skills in a modern, high-tech environment. Add to that the amazing teaching staff and our in-depth clinical experiences and you have a recipe for success in the real world. I was amazed by how much my education impacted the care I gave every day when I started working as a bedside nurse at Caromont Health. My clinical instructor's voice rang in my head each day as I approached different situations and remembered to apply all of my knowledge, practical skills, and critical thinking ability.

During nursing school, I was a member of the ANS—the Association of Nursing Students. The group underwent a revival during my time in nursing school and became a thriving organization with a focus on community service and outreach, as well as founding a memorial scholarship in honor of Ashley Lutz, a senior nursing student who passed away after receiving her pin in May 2011.

As a student, I was fortunate enough to be selected by faculty to serve as a student liaison to the SON Alumni Chapter, eventually becoming a full-fledged member at graduation and having the honor of serving as president for a two-year term.

I could not be more grateful for the education I received at UNC Charlotte School of Nursing, and for my experience with the School of Nursing Alumni Chapter. I look forward to growing in my career and as an active alumnus, continuing to be an active part of the community and a part of the next chapter in UNC Charlotte School of Nursing history.

JANIS JOYCE, MSN, RN, CLASS OF 2009[3]

When I first began to think about completing my MSN, it seemed like a dream. I don't know why I had not considered pursuing an advanced degree. I guess I always thought it was for academic nurses. However, the more I read about what it meant for a nurse to be able to say she had a master's the more I felt it was something I wanted to do. I applied in 2005 and was accepted to begin my journey in 2006. During my three years of study, our country experienced economic crises with the housing market, banking, and the auto industry. I began to understand how my master's was going to make me a more valuable nurse. As a more valuable nurse, my options increased dramatically. This was a comforting thought, even though I had never had a problem getting a job, the possibility was a sobering one.

In the midst of pursing my degree, I accepted a job that required I commute weekly to Wilmington, Delaware. In years past, I would have had to delay my education until my consulting job was over. However, due to the online program that was offered by UNC Charlotte, I was able to continue uninterrupted. I can remember being so appreciative of the "new" way of learning. I admit to being skeptical at first because I had never participated in online classes before then. I was pleasantly surprised to find that my learning was probably more intense because I had to communicate my opinions for each assignment rather than just show up for a class and not say a word. I was charged with "presenting my case" on each topic in a class. The challenge was empowering. I learned I could be eloquent and passionate about topics that I had a particular interest in and I learned that others could be just as passionate when they disagreed. This really was a growth experience for me in not just my education, but in my communication. I had already been a nurse for more than 20 years and it had been 10 years since I had completed my BSN. I had forgotten how much I enjoyed the academic world. I met new friends. I was able to participate in a study abroad in The Netherlands, Germany, and Belgium. While in Europe, I had an asthma flare-up, so I got to really experience the medical system from a firsthand perspective. I was very pleased with how I was treated and how efficient the system worked. It offered an "ah ha" moment when I thought about how nervous I had been about having to seek medical treatment in a country in which I did not speak the language. My experience could not have been better; but, it could have been different if the people caring for me had not tried to understand me, had been unkind to me, or had not shown clinical expertise. I thought about the rising number of patients we care for in our country who don't speak English and are most likely experiencing the same anxious feelings when they have to seek medical care in our country. I use the kindness shown to me as a model for how I want to treat all people, and I am more sensitive to cultural diversity since that experience.

During the last year of my program, I accepted a new job as a nurse manager of an inpatient post-operative unit. Additionally, I had a life-threatening anaphylactic reaction about six months before the end of my degree and ended up in the ICU for a couple of nights. This occurred during our tri-annual Joint Commission Survey. My mother became critically ill around this same time. All in all, looking back, I can honestly say this was one of the most difficult and intense years of my life. But, boy, did it feel great when I finished that master's!!!

My UNC Charlotte School of Nursing journey not only increased my knowledge, but also helped me grow as a person. I credit the professors for their commitment to excellence in nursing education. I had a great experience and am so glad I made the decision to go back to school when I did. My husband tells me all the time how proud he is of my accomplishments. I am proud, too.

JACKIE DIENEMANN, CHAIR OF ADULT HEALTH, 2003–2006, AND FACULTY, 2007–2010[4]

I came to live in Davidson in 2000. At that time, there was a hiring freeze for state employees. First, I was hired by Safe Alliance from a grant to assess the need for a DV Hospital Program at Carolinas Medical Center. This led to creation of the DVHP program. Then, at the request of Dr. Bill Cody and Dean Bishop at the College of Health Professions, I was hired to work with the Health Department to identify healthcare needs for the homeless. This led to the Homeless Healthcare Alliance that identified priorities for this population in the community, and over time, these have been met. Meanwhile, I taught part time in the Nursing Department and the Office of Research for the College.

In 2003, I was asked to become the chair of Adult Health (undergraduate courses in Adult Health, MSN in FNP, ANP/CNS, CRNA, Nursing Administration, and MSN/MHA) when the current chair left abruptly. I was told that this was a disorganized group with low morale. I accepted. I had no experience with acute care (the focus of this department), so I met with faculty and told them I would be reliant on their specialty expertise. We met monthly, and over time, morale improved. I led curriculum changes to the MSN in FNP, separating the ANP and Acute Care CNS, updating the PMHCNS, and adding a MSN in Education to the Community Health CNS. The ANP/CNS program was deleted. The Synthesis capstone course was rethought to have students apply what they had learned about research or EBP by working with faculty to support their research or doing EBP projects with MSN-prepared nurses in practice settings. All students presented a poster on their work at a professional meeting. In 2004–05, I was chair of the committee to establish an interdisciplinary PhD in Health Sciences research. It was approved and, in 2005, began as the first PhD in the college. I was active in the Health Services Research Council and later was president.

Meanwhile, in 2005, Dean Bishop retired and the colleges were reorganized. The College of Health and Human Services was created with a School of Nursing and departments of Public Health, Social Work, and Kinesiology. During that time, I was able to support Dr. Hardin to do a post doc at UNC Chapel Hill. This was part of our efforts to increase research productivity in nursing. The SON faculty had received an R21 (Judith Cornelius), and several faculty were publishing and beginning to expand programs of research.

In 2006, the school was reorganized without chairs and the MSN/MHA, Psychiatric-MH CNS, and Acute Care CNS MSNs were inactivated. Dr. Cody, who had been the Family Health chair, left. I continued to serve on multiple committees but was no longer in an administrative role. During that time, my greatest contribution was to support Dr. Coffman to apply and receive a Robert Woods Johnson Faculty Scholars appointment (equivalent to a post doc). I also assisted several faculty in the college who left to make positive career changes. I did research with Marcia Shobe and Shanti Kukami in social work and supported Shanti to attain tenure. I also did research with the Mecklenburg County Women's Commission to refine the Domestic Violence Survivor Assessment.

In 2008, I served on the early planning committee of the joint post-master's DNP with WCU. This grew out of my leading an application for a HRSA grant to strengthen the Nursing Administration MSN that we did not receive but WCU did receive. The original plan was to have the first DNP in the state, but the state wanted to simultaneously start DNPs at multiple UNC universities.

Since retirement, I have worked with Sigma Theta Tau as the research chair, served on the DV Advisory Board for the city/county, been active in NCNA, acted as a consultant to a PhD program in New York, and continued to work part time for Carolinas Healthcare System to mentor nurses in evidence-based practice and research.

SHARON R. ALLEN, MSN, RN-BC, CDE, CNE, DNP STUDENT

MSN in Nursing Education, May 2013

When I graduated with my BSN in 1984, I always wanted to do my master's degree in nursing. After almost 15 years of missionary nursing in Ecuador, we returned to the U.S. and settled in Charlotte. UNC Charlotte was close to our home, so it was wonderful to have an excellent university nearby where I could study.

Health Disparities was one of the core courses I took for the online MSN in nursing education. Dr. Maren Coffman taught this course in a very thought-provoking manner and I was able to apply my life experiences with Latinos in the course. Because of our similar life work with Spanish speakers, Dr. Coffman and I had an instant connection. Later, I was her teacher's assistant on a trip to Costa Rica to observe and evaluate the Costa Rican healthcare system. Then when it was time to do my synthesis project, Dr. Coffman was a phenomenal guide as we did research with technology (fitbit pedometers) with women at a local free clinic.

After graduation, with the MSN in nursing education in 2013, Dr. Coffman invited me to go with her to present our research (via poster presentation) in 2014 at the Southern Nursing Research Society. She has always been an encourager and help to me and is now a committee member for my DNP in Nursing Education Capstone Project as I continue to work with technology (text messaging) with Latinos at a Free Clinic in Charlotte.

Dr. Lienne Edwards has been an encourager and guide to me, and asked me to return to UNC Charlotte to teach in the BSN program. Since 2014 I have been adjunct faculty teaching courses on campus in the BSN program, online in the RN-BSN program, and this fall in the online MSN program. I am grateful for the excellent master's-level nursing education I received at UNC Charlotte and am now honored to pass along this education to nursing students in the UNC Charlotte SON undergraduate and graduate programs.

Pictures of Students through the Years
(Note how the uniform changes.)

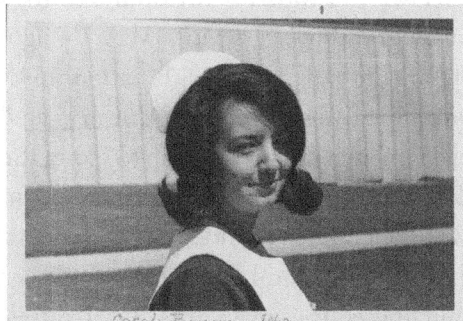

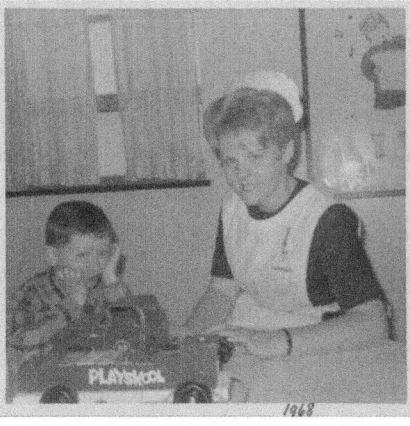

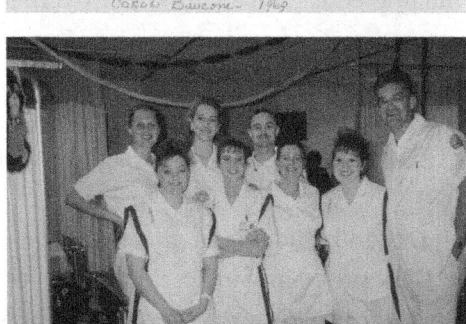

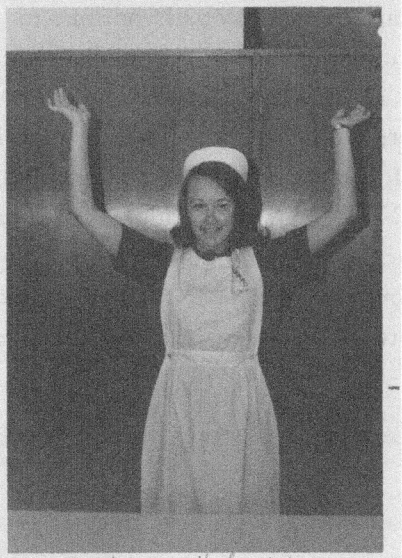

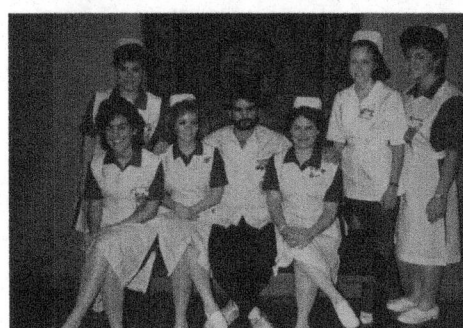

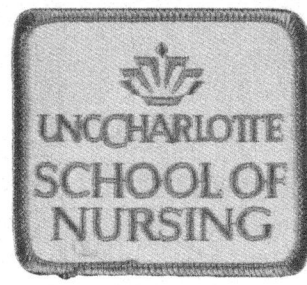

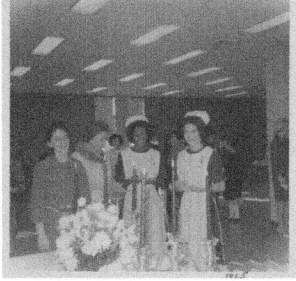

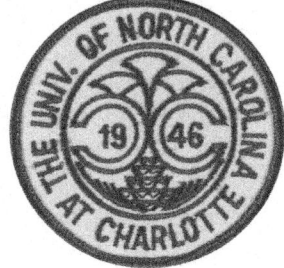

Nursing uniform collage.

CHAPTER ELEVEN

Beyond the Classroom

Dona Haney, RN, MSN
UNC Charlotte Nursing Alumni Interest Group

In late 1976, a group of nursing alumni began discussing the possibility of creating an organization. They felt that nursing alumni would be interested in following events at the College of Nursing and what classmates were doing. A task force was formed. The participants were:

Beth Alexander (class of '68)
Dona Haney (class of '69)
Lynn Dobson (class of '70)
Sue Head (class of '71)
Glenna Davenport-Cook (class of '72)
Sherry Heine (class of '73)
Patty Lawrence (class of '74)
Diane Helms Benedict (class of '75)
Betsy McLean (1976)
Susan Piscitelli, director of Alumni Affairs

The organization of the UNC Charlotte Nursing Alumni Interest Group would take place within the framework of the University General Alumni Association. The proposed objectives were to

- maintain communications and relationships among nursing alumni,
- provide visibility for UNC Charlotte's College of Nursing in the Charlotte community,
- add input into the direction to be taken by the College of Nursing,
- supply information about college and university services,

- create a support system for new graduates by making them aware of job opportunities, etc., and
- encourage maintenance of the high professional standards already demonstrated by the College of Nursing.

The work of organizing and motivating the alumni began and Dona Haney, BSN, class of '69 was asked to be the first president of the group.

By the spring of 1978, the 10th anniversary of the first graduating class, the group planned a meeting to be held in conjunction with the Sigma Theta Tau Spring Luncheon and Lecture. The agenda for that meeting included a brief overview of the College of Nursing activities from Dean Louise Schlachter; a tribute to Chancellor Dean Colvard who was retiring; a report on the status of the UNC Charlotte Chapter of Sigma Theta Tau Honor Society for Nursing; a report of the many Continuing Education offerings; and the election of officers, board members, and class representatives.

By the third annual meeting of the Nursing Alumni Interest Group in 1979, members had established the Edith Brocker Award; and through the efforts of the class representatives, they had prepared the first *News Notes,* a bulletin that provided updates on individual alumni.

The Edith Brocker Award was created in honor of the College of Nursing's first dean. With her assistance, it was decided that an award be created to honor a graduating student for her or his professional contribution, leadership, and scholastic achievement. The award was given for the first time in 1979 to Robin Sink (Deal).

A subsequent issue of the *News Notes* included

- updates on the lives and careers of 71 alumni from the classes of 1969–1978,
- a report from Donna Bumgarner Nussman on the success of the Sigma Theta Tau chapter, established in 1978, now with 230 members, and
- a report by Betsy Mclean describing the Edith Brocker Award being given to Patricia Powell,[1] and a new Teacher of Excellence Award that had been given in September 1980 to Vera Smith. It was noted that Vera was one of the early faculty. "For the first few years, she, along with two others, taught all the courses to all the students. Vera's greatest strength was one of being a student advocate. Vera has meant so much to so many of us. Thank you, Vera, for teaching us how to live."[2]

The last documentation of the Nursing Alumni Interest Group meeting is an invitation to the 1980 Spring Meeting by President Betsy McLean. The meeting was scheduled to occur the morning before the Fifth Annual Luncheon and Lecture. The speaker at the luncheon was Sister Rosemary Donley, dean of the School of Nursing, Catholic University of America, Washington, DC. Her topic for the keynote address was "Health Policy Strategies at State and National Levels."

Although the Nursing Alumni Interest Group ceased activity, the faculty continued to give the Edith Brocker Award each year at graduation.

UNC Charlotte School of Nursing Alumni Chapter (SONAC)

In 2010, the first academic alumni chapter of the UNC Charlotte campus was founded, and it was the School of Nursing Alumni Chapter (SONAC). The beginning of this chapter should be credited to Dr. Dee Baldwin. Details of the founding of this chapter are based on conversations with Dr. Baldwin (known to alumni as "Dee") as well as some early documentation in the archives of the Atkins Library.

Dr. Baldwin became associate dean and director of the School of Nursing in 2009. When she arrived, she spent time meeting nurses and alumni in the community. She commented that many alumni "were doing great things," but she did not see a connection between alumni and the university, and believed that the university did not "do enough" to recognize publicly the accomplishments of the alumni.[3]

Dr. Baldwin began meeting informally at the university Starbucks with Heather Shaughnessy, director of Development for the College of Health and Human Services, and Chip Rossi, director of Alumni Affairs for the University, to discuss possibilities. She describes the three of them as "The Three-legged Stool" and their meetings as "great fun." Shaughnessy noted that many of the significant donors to the university were nursing alumni, and many of the scholarships within the college were donated by nursing alumni. Rossi was trying to strengthen the alumni association at the university level, and the three worked together hoping to re-engage and re-energize alumni.

In June 2010, a large group of nursing alumni received a notice that Alumni Affairs, in partnership with the School of Nursing, would be establishing a School of Nursing Alumni Chapter. They were invited "to guide the formation of this group by attending an upcoming social and focus group."[4] Two sessions were scheduled, one in the early afternoon, and one in the evening. Both sessions were well attended. After hearing the overall plan, individuals willing to be founding board members of the School of Nursing Alumni Chapter (SONAC) signed up to participate. At the first board meeting, Dona Haney was elected to be the first president of UNC Charlotte SONAC. Other officers elected were J. R. Hildreth, vice-president, and Bunny Eubanks, secretary.

The group spent much of their time discussing what would entice alumni to become involved as well as how they could encourage students to become involved after graduation. A student, Aly Bell, was invited to become a part of the group and was so instrumental that she would become SONAC's second president. By 2011, SONAC had established its first project, the SONAC Emergency Fund. Ann Newman, an alumna who had been on the faculty for many years had suggested that often students needed funds on an emergency basis to continue the semester or move on to the next semester. Thus, the SONAC Emergency Fund was "established to assist nursing students with the most critical financial needs due to unforeseen hardships or unanticipated events." The fund provided a one-time award of up to $500 toward tuition and fees. The organization has had requests for these funds almost each year.

SONAC's second major project came to fruition in 2012. The group felt that alumni would value a continuing education opportunity (with continuing education credits), a class by an outstanding speaker or leader. Along with an educational focus, the team designed the Nursing Distinguished Alumni Award that would be presented as a part of the event, thus the Distinguished Alumni Nursing Lectureship was born.

The first lectureship focused on healthcare reform; the speaker was Mayra Alvarez, director of Public Health Policy Office of Health Reform, U.S. Department of Health and Human Services. The conference was sponsored by the Carolinas Medical Center and UNC Charlotte, under the leadership of Bill Leonard, president of Carolinas Medical Center University. Our first Distinguished Alumni Award went to Lynda C. Opdyke, RN, MSN.

The second week of February became the traditional time for our Distinguished Alumni Lectureship. The award was supported by the university and Leonard. So far, six individuals have received the title of Distinguished Alumni.

In 2015, SONAC awarded our first School of Nursing Honorary Nursing Alumni award, an award for an individual who is not an alumnus of the school, to Elinor B. Caddell, RN, MSN, a founding member of the university's faculty, who had a long, distinguished career at UNC Charlotte. Faculty and alumni nominated Caddell for this award. Although she retired in 1989, she continues to be a resource to alumni and provides a scholarship to assist faculty with research.

SONAC is excited to be a part of the 50th anniversary celebration of the School of Nursing. We look forward to being a part of the next 50 years.

Sigma Theta Tau at UNC Charlotte, Gamma Iota Chapter
Dona Haney, RN, MSN

Even before the UNC Charlotte College of Nursing Gamma Iota Chapter of Sigma Theta Tau was officially chartered, Dean Marinell Jernigan and faculty initiated a Nursing Honor Society. In March 1978, the Nursing Honor Society of UNC Charlotte's College of Nursing became officially chartered as the Gamma Iota Chapter of Sigma Theta Tau.

Membership in Sigma Theta Tau is an honor conferred on students in baccalaureate and graduate programs who have demonstrated excellence in their programs. Graduates of baccalaureate programs who demonstrate excellence in leadership positions in nursing are also eligible for consideration. Membership applications are invited from those who excel in scholastic achievement, community involvement, and peer evaluation.

The founding officers of the Gamma Iota Chapter were:

President: Judith H. Grubbs
Vice-President: Elizabeth D. McLean
Corresponding Secretary: Belinda S. Worsham
Recording Secretary: Beth W. Lindsay
Treasurer: Robin H. Lee
Archivist: Susan K. Willis
Faculty: Marinell H. Jernigan, Susan S. Harvey

The initial inductees included 101 new members with 12 faculty and community members transferring in. The transfers included:

Raymond A. Andrews, Beta Omicron
Alice B. Barrington, Alpha Alpha
Kay K. Chitty, Alpha Epsilon
Sandra F. Goble, Pi
Susan S. Harvey, Alpha Alpha
Sue G. Head, Alpha Alpha
Marinell Jernigan, Nu
Shirley A. Kotlarz, Alpha Epsilon
Casmira Marciniszyn, Xi
Ruth N. Mauldin, Nu
Sally Nicholson, Alpha Alpha
Marilyn G. Smith, Alpha Alpha
Laurie Wilshire, Beta Pi

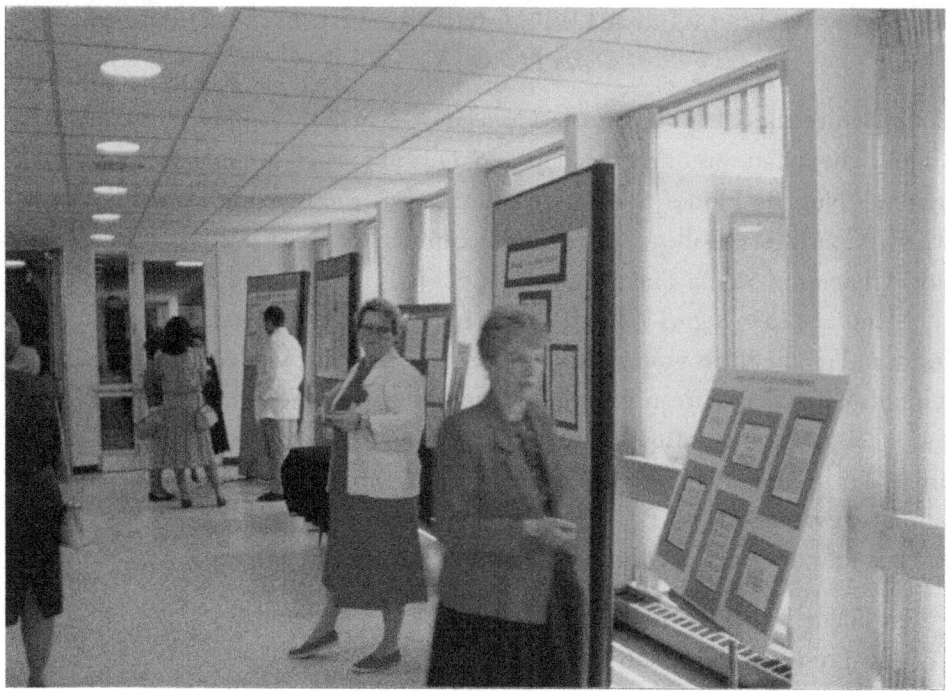

Dr. Kay Boggs and Dr. Barbara Carper review Research Posters
at Sigma Theta Tau Research Day, 1996.

Gamma Iota's Spring Lectureship and Luncheon quickly took its place as an annual event at the College of Nursing. National nursing leaders were invited to present and Miss Bonnie always attended the event, which was co-sponsored by the College of Nursing and Gamma Iota. As the chapter grew, a Research Day was added and continues to be an important part of student learning. By faculty sharing the research they engaged in, they role modeled for students the importance of research in their practice.

Currently there are 220 active members in the campus chapter. The chapter has grown since its inception and has gained recognition for overall excellence. On two occasions, it was awarded outstanding national awards known as chapter key awards in 1993 and 1995 for their efforts in attaining chapter goals. In addition to the annual Research Day, other activities have included participating in a walk-a-thon, raising awareness and collecting donations for the local women's shelter, providing funding to support local community services such as the homeless shelter, and offering stress relievers for current School of Nursing students such as chocolate bars and Starbucks coffee cards during exam week.

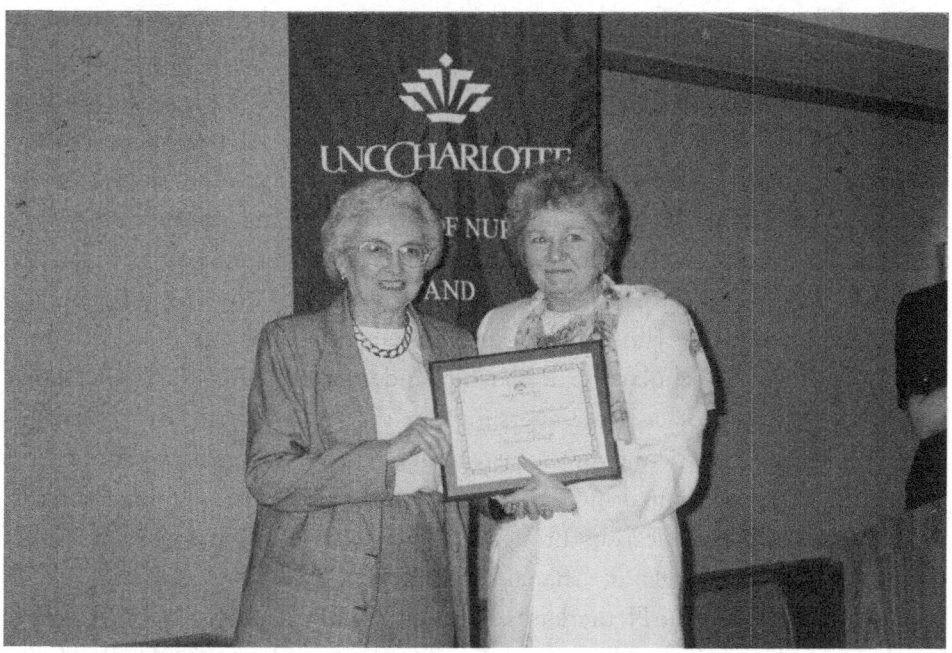

Elinor Caddell, founder of the Elinor Brooks Caddell Faculty Scholar Award,
announced at the Gamma Iota Spring Lectureship by Dean Bishop, 1996.

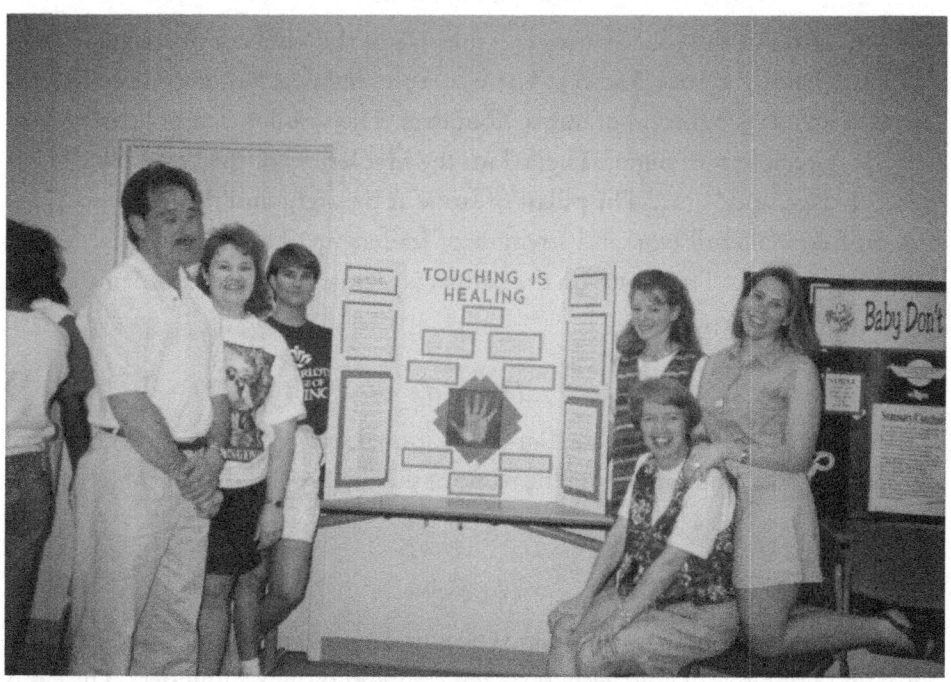

Senior students present their research.

Sigma Theta Tau was founded in 1922 by six students at the University Training School for Nurses in Indianapolis, Indiana. The name was chosen using the initials of the three Greek words "storga," "tharos," and "tima," meaning love, courage, and honor. Sigma Theta Tau was organized to encourage and recognize superior scholastic and leadership achievement at the undergraduate and graduate levels in nursing. Sigma Theta Tau is a member of the Association of College Honor Societies and is professional and scholarly, rather than social, in its purposes.

The Sigma Theta Tau International Honor Society of Nursing (Sigma), is a nonprofit organization whose mission is advancing world health and celebrating nursing excellence in scholarship, leadership, and service. Founded in 1922, Sigma has more than 135,000 active members in more than 90 countries and territories. Members include practicing nurses, instructors, researchers, policymakers, entrepreneurs, and others. Sigma's more than 530 chapters are located at more than 700 institutions of higher education throughout Armenia, Australia, Botswana, Brazil, Canada, Colombia, England, Ghana, Hong Kong, Japan, Jordan, Kenya, Lebanon, Malawi, Mexico, the Netherlands, Pakistan, Philippines, Portugal, Singapore, South Africa, South Korea, Swaziland, Sweden, Taiwan, Tanzania, Thailand, the United States, and Wales.[5]

The Coat of Arms

The symbolism of the coat of arms is expressive of the ideals of this Sigma Theta Tau International Honor Society. The eye represents wisdom and discernment. The stars are in recognition of our six founders. The scroll is that of learning and bears the Greek letters, Sigma Theta Tau: the first letters of the Greek words "storgé," "tharsos, and "timé." The pillars of stone at the right and the left denote service, professional endeavor, and strength of leadership. The lamp represents the lamp of knowledge. The motto on the banner is Sigma Theta Tau, the name of this international honor society.[6]

The Seal

The imprint of the Sigma Theta Tau International seal is the lamp of knowledge surrounded by a circle containing the name of the society and the date of its founding, 1922.[7]

The Key

The key is the symbol of scholarship. The cup denotes the satisfaction of professional life. The circle of gold with its six stars represents our six founders. The lamp

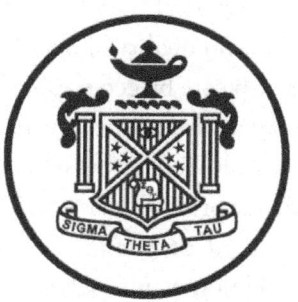

Sigma Theta Tau
International coat of arms.

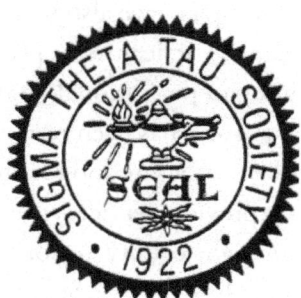

Sigma Theta Tau
International seal.

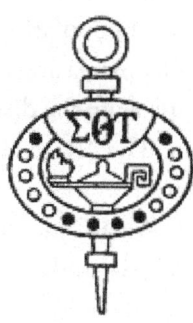

Sigma Theta Tau
International key.

is the lamp of knowledge. The letters in black—Sigma Theta Tau—represent our charge of storgé, tharsos, timé or love, courage, honor.[8]

UNC Charlotte and AHEC: Growing Together
Yuen L. Cheung (May), MSN, RN-BC

This year, UNC Charlotte School of Nursing (SON) is celebrating its 50th anniversary, and the North Carolina Area Health Education Centers (NC AHEC) is celebrating its 45th anniversary. I was asked to write an article about UNC Charlotte SON and NC AHEC to commemorate these two momentous occasions. In order to better understand the relationship between UNC Charlotte School of Nursing and AHEC, I reached out to Dona Haney, president of the UNC Charlotte SON Alumni Association. Dona brought me to the archives in the J. Murrey Atkins Library. I spent a couple of afternoons at the library reviewing archived documents that detailed the achievements of both institutions. I came to realize that the relationship between NC AHEC and UNC Charlotte SON has roots that go back four decades.

In 1972, UNC Chapel Hill (UNC) was awarded an $8.5 million federal contract to help develop Area Health Education Centers across the state. This funding helped create three centers including the AHEC in Charlotte. In 1974, state funding enabled UNC to add six additional centers to adequately serve all regions of the state.

NC AHEC's goal has always been to provide continuing professional development programs and services that bridge academic institutions and communities to improve the health of the people of North Carolina with a focus on the underserved population. The centers have also met the state's health and workforce needs by increasing the quantity of healthcare providers and quality of health care by improving the distribution of professionals and health care by geographical location. The NC AHEC's mission has been to regionalize professional healthcare education as well, in hopes of attracting and retaining healthcare professionals.

NC AHEC in Charlotte provides services to healthcare professionals and health professions students in an eight-county region composed of Anson, Cabarrus, Cleveland, Gaston, Lincoln, Mecklenburg, Stanly, and Union counties. Leadership in the Charlotte AHEC included Dr. Bryant Galusha, director of NC AHEC, and Marcia Brooks, RN, MSN, coordinator of Nursing Education, both were very involved with UNC Charlotte School of Nursing in planning collaborative initiatives.

From 1974–80, NC AHEC funded the UNC Charlotte Outreach master's program at UNC Chapel Hill. This program allowed students from the Charlotte area to commute to Chapel Hill for course work. Funding provided the transportation to and from Chapel Hill for weekly classes. Funds also supported faculty involvement for student training in clinical experiences provided by NC AHEC through a contract with the Charlotte AHEC.

UNC Charlotte also partnered with NC AHEC in Asheville to provide access to the graduate program for baccalaureate-prepared nurses residing in the far western part of the state. This was done by combining televised classes originating in Charlotte and onsite clinical experiences in Asheville. It was an efficient use of resources and required only a part-time supervisor for the clinical practicum in Asheville. Additionally, the nursing director at the Asheville AHEC location sat in on every class as it was televised in order to assure the transmission and reception was smooth and effective. In 1988–89, 28 students were enrolled in this outreach program.

In 1989, the North Carolina General Assembly provided funding to NC AHEC to create innovative programs in partnership with North Carolina schools of nursing. Three key initiatives were established: a statewide registered nurse refresher program, clinical site development grants, and educational mobility programs for registered nurses to move on to BSN and MSN degrees. To this day, funding supports these nursing initiatives.

Since its inception, the Charlotte AHEC has often partnered with local experts on the UNC Charlotte SON faculty to teach continuing nursing education programs, such as the nurse educator's certification preparation course and the nursing faculty development course for practicing nurses and nurse educators. UNC Charlotte SON also receives funding from the NC AHEC program to develop new clinical sites and nursing programs.

Congratulations to UNC Charlotte SON for reaching its 50-year milestone. The NC AHEC and Charlotte AHEC are looking forward to our continued partnership and future collaborations.

Reaching into the Community
Margaret M. "Peggy" Patton, MSN, MSEd, RN

Nurses have long recognized the need to utilize their skills and to serve not only in a clinical setting, but in the larger community as well. Nurses provide skilled care to patients and families in the short term when acute illness or injury presents, but nursing's long-range goal is to help individuals help themselves. "Meet the client where he is," has long been the mantra of nurses in community outreach programs. They teach and equip mothers to bring healthier babies into the world, parents to care for their families, older adults to care for themselves, and adult children to care for their aging parents.

This need for community outreach was recognized by UNC Charlotte's administration and the School of Nursing early in the school's history, and its practices and programs have grown with the city of Charlotte. Faculty have shared this passion for community service with their students through instruction in family-oriented nursing care. Providing instruction in health care, education in disease prevention. and health promotions is only part of the picture. Nursing has actively searched for the underserved and provided innovative solutions to answer their unmet needs.

In 1989, as the School of Nursing was growing and seeking increasing clinical learning exposures for the students, faculty members found an unmet need—homeless women and children. Three nursing faculty from UNC Charlotte SON had been volunteering at the George Shinn Center for homeless men, when they realized that homeless women and children did not have the same access to health care. When a mother is struggling to put a roof over her babies' heads and give them something to eat, she may not be thinking about when they had their last immunizations or how to get rid of that nasty little cold. The Salvation Army of Hope on Spratt Street in Charlotte had a shelter for homeless women and their children, but no health care. Oftentimes, women experiencing such profoundly competing priorities as shelter, food, and employment find it difficult or impossible to balance those needs with care for their children who are most often with them instead of their fathers. The clinic at the men's shelter had remarkably improved the men's health. So, the faculty members—Marilyn Smith, Lynn Dobson, and Emily Chiles—approached the Salvation Army about setting up a clinic for these women and children. The project was approved and began in 1989.

The clinic was set up in a corner of the dayroom because all of the women tended to spend some time there. At first, their new clients were suspicious. "We sat there, with our borrowed stethoscopes, and sort of said, 'OK, here we are . . . when you're ready,'" Dobson recalled. "Gradually, they began to come to us."[9] During clinic time, which was three hours one afternoon a week, the nurses saw a wide range of problems. They found that the women and children were not as acutely ill as the men, who experienced severe substance abuse problems and long-term diseases brought on and exacerbated by poor living conditions and health behaviors. The women were healthier and trying to make sure their children were as well.

"Otherwise, their needs were no different from anyone else's," Chiles said.[10] The children came to the clinic for all of the usual needs: upper respiratory infections, immunizations, and ear infections. The women came for issues related to pregnancy and information about Pap smears. The nurses and volunteers provided care and education about maintaining good health. Smith says that she and the others believed in nursing as community health care and education, not just "putting a patient in a room and taking vital signs."[11]

At times, the clinic staff referred patients who required more care than they could provide. These referrals and advocacy on the part of the clinic staff was important in getting these patients, who were "outside of the system," the care they needed. Their patients were able to have their needs fully met before they became acute.

In addition to delivering the only health care that most of these women and children received, the clinic provided hands-on training for students in the bachelor of science in nursing and master of science in nursing programs. This was invaluable clinical experience for students in direct nursing care and in the study of sociological and psychological causes and effects of community healthcare problems in vulnerable populations. Nearly every semester saw a steady rotation of third- and fourth-year students, as well as graduate students in community health and nurse practitioner programs. The shelter residents who used the clinic commented often on how much they enjoyed interacting with the eager and enthusiastic students.

Toward the end of the 1990s, Dr. William K. Cody, chair of the Family and Community Nursing Department in the School of Nursing, became the faculty member responsible for overseeing the clinic. Under Dr. Cody's oversight, the clinic grew in the area it occupied at the Salvation Army and in the numbers that it served. Dr. Cody also helped fund the clinic with fundraising events and grants. The grants greatly improved the services of the clinic, allowing them to hire a nurse and an administrative assistant to manage clinic services and referrals.

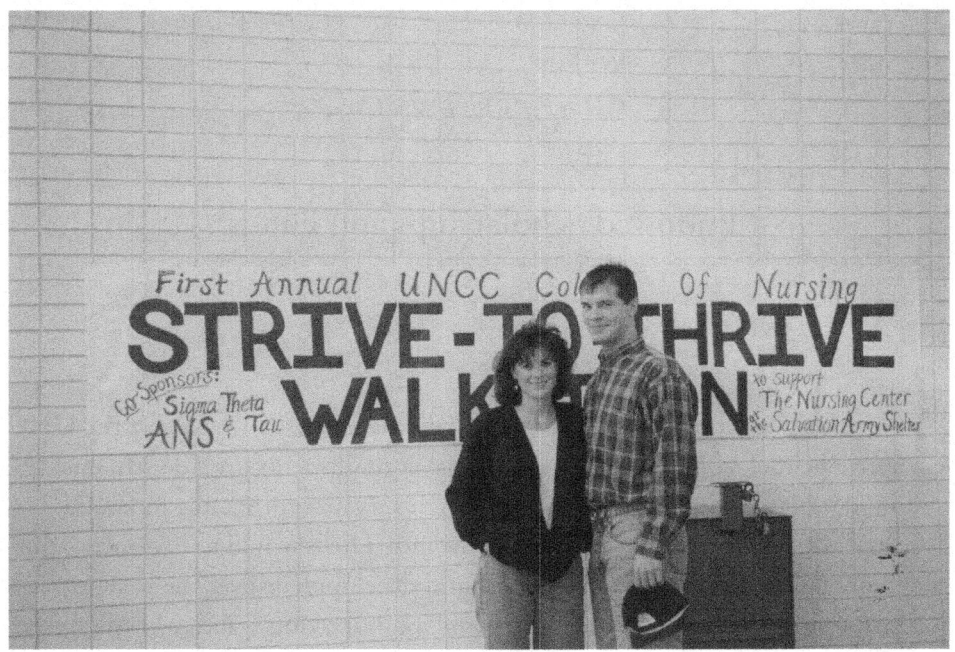

Nursing students fundraising for the Salvation Army shelter.

Numerous Charlotte-area physicians volunteered their time and medical skills to the clinic. With increased funding, some were paid small stipends for their participation. The clinic also used volunteer nurse practitioners. All of these healthcare professionals provided high-level care to a segment of the population that would have gone otherwise without.

During its sixteenth year, in July 2005, the clinic, now called the Uptown Clinic, changed its administrative design, staffing structure, and principle income source. UNC Charlotte SON would no longer support the clinic, which had grown into the largest medical and nursing clinic for homeless people in Charlotte. Shelter Health Services, Inc., became the clinic's new name. The location, mission, and services remained the same. Funding became totally dependent on private grants and fundraising. Volunteer physicians, nurses, and nurse practitioners continued to provide care, while overall management of the clinic was transferred from Dr. Cody to Michelle Carr, the nurse who had been head of nursing services at the clinic. Cody became chair of the newly formed board of directors.

Services to this deserving and vulnerable population were begun by nurses who saw a need and acted on that need with the cooperation of the Salvation Army. Services to these mothers and their children continue.

CHAPTER TWELVE

Endowed Scholarships and Funds[1]

We are greatly indebted to the individuals who have chosen to support the UNC Charlotte School of Nursing. Their financial commitments provide scholarships, endowed professorships, and endowed funds that support programs and initiatives. Without the generosity of our donors, some individuals would not be able to pursue their educations, the school's growth and development over the past 50 years would not have been as profound, nor would we be looking as such a bright future. The following awards have been funded by, or given in honor of, the individuals named.

James R. (J.R.) and Donna Gregory Hildreth Scholarship
Ruth C. Clarke Scholarship
Dean W. Colvard Distinguished Professor in Nursing
Carol Grotnes Belk Endowed Chair in Nursing
Nursing Alumni Scholarship Endowment
Artie Sue Kerley Professorship in Nursing
Penny R. Thomas Memorial Scholarship Fund
Elinor Brooks Caddell Faculty Award
Piedmont Club Foundation Nursing Scholarship
Agnes Binder Weisiger Nursing Scholarship
Bronna Hackney Nursing Endowment
John and Alice Harney Endowment
Emerald Care Home Health Nursing Scholarship
William D. and Nancy B. Thomas Scholarship for Nursing
Ann Mabe Newman and William G. Newman Endowed Nursing Scholarship
Jim and Nancy Hill Scholarship Fund
Professor Carol P. Fray Student Endowed Scholarship
Newman Interaction Labs
Prof. Frances R. King Nursing Scholarship

William Randolph Hearst Endowed Scholarship
Marilyn Greene Smith Learning Laboratory Endowment Fund
Alice E. Mazarick Scholarship in Nursing
Ashley Lutz Memorial Scholarship Fund
Beverly B. Horton Memorial Scholarship Fund

CHAPTER THIRTEEN

Named Areas within the College of Nursing[1]

The following areas of the college are named for faculty who had outstanding careers and made major contributions to the College of Nursing.

Dr. Sue Marquis Bishop Auditorium

Sue Bishop, PhD, served as the dean and professor in the College of Health and Human Services from 1992–2004. She was respected and admired by her faculty and her colleagues, both on- and off-campus. She was instrumental in leading the college through the transition from the College of Nursing to the College of Nursing and Health Professions to the present College of Health and Human Services. Under her leadership, the college developed many programs to meet the nursing shortage, broadened its offerings in health and human services disciplines, and created a research environment in a multidisciplinary atmosphere. She positioned the college's move to a doctoral/research-intensive college. She was also instrumental in defining needs and spaces for the college in its new building.

The Director of the School of Nursing's Suite: Elinor Caddell

Elinor Caddell, RN, MSN, was an extremely well-prepared nurse who had worked with Dean Edith Brocker at Duke University prior to being offered the position of the first faculty member in the UNC Charlotte Department of Nursing. She remained for 24 years, progressing from assistant professor to professor. She was nominated for a number of prestigious awards and was recognized as a pioneer in nursing education. Caddell was instrumental in establishing the curricula and other preparatory materials the school needed to be accredited as a master's of nursing institution. With a commitment to supporting life-long learning, she founded the Elinor Caddell Faculty Research Award. Caddell was awarded the Honorary Alumnus Award from the University of North Carolina at Charlotte Alumni as well as the School of Nursing Alumni.

Marilyn Greene Smith Living Learning Lab

Marilyn Smith, MSN, started her teaching career as an instructor in nursing at the University of North Carolina at Charlotte in 1977 after receiving her BSN from UNC Charlotte in 1971. In July 1989 with collaboration of fellow faculty member Emily Chiles, MSN, RN, they founded and staffed the Nursing Clinic at the Salvation Army for Women and Children. She completed her Family Nurse Practitioner course while teaching at UNC Charlotte in 1993. She became a certified Sexual Assault Nurse Examiner in 2002 and a certified Forensic Nurse Examiner in 2003. An anonymous former student donated the Marilyn Greene Smith Learning Center in her honor. Greene retired in 2008.

Ann Mabe and William G. Newman Interaction Lab

Ann M. Newman, PhD, came to the UNC Charlotte School of Nursing as an RN seeking a BSN. She was a student representative on the new Pathways program. Thus began her leadership role at the School of Nursing. Immediately upon graduating from the BSN, she pursued a MSN in the new collaborative program between UNC Chapel Hill and UNC Charlotte. Upon graduation, she began a distinguished career at the UNC Charlotte School of Nursing where she taught for 34 years, focusing on mental health and leadership. Her commendations and awards have been numerous, including the first Elinor Caddell Faculty Scholarship, the Bank of America Teacher of Excellence, and the Distinguished Alumni Award. Upon the death of her beloved husband, William Gray Newman, she endowed the Interaction Lab.

CHAPTER FOURTEEN

Research and Scholarship

Jacqueline Dienemann, RN, PH, FAAN

UNC Charlotte, the College of Health and Human Services, and then the School of Nursing was first envisioned as a teaching institution. Over time it grew and so did the programs it provided, including master's programs. By the 1980s, scholarship and research became a newly emerging focus. The first step under Dean Nancy Langston, RN, PhD, was to encourage faculty to publish articles that reported on the school's service and clinical practice activities. The school began to build infrastructure to support publishing by hiring a consultant to assist in editing and submitting manuscripts. Faculty, who chose to return for their doctorates, were encouraged and supported. The school also sought new faculty with doctoral degrees. By 1989, one manuscript had been published in a refereed journal; the following year, there were six.

The school was successful in recruiting new doctorally prepared faculty and supporting those who chose to return to earn new doctorates. In 1989, 10 of 32 faculty members had doctorates, and by 1991 there were 23. In 1993, Sue Bishop, RN, PhD, became dean of the College of Nursing. In 1994, Elinor Brooks Caddell, RN, MSN, endowed a fund for an annual grant to a faculty member to support a research project. The Gamma Iota Chapter of Sigma Theta Tau at UNC Charlotte offered competitive grants annually. These two ongoing grants nurtured the faculty as they grew their research. In 1993, the school established the first Research Colloquium for faculty to report on their research to their peers.

In 1995, the university was restructured to create a College of Nursing and Health Professions with a School of Nursing, Department of Social Work, and Department of Health Promotion and Kinesiology. In 1996, the Office of Nursing and Health Research was begun by Dean Bishop. Debra Hymovich, RN, PhD, was appointed to be the first associate dean for Research. She had been working half time as the director of Research since 1994 and had assisted in strengthening resources for the College of Nursing and building confidence in grant administration.

In 1995, the school received a $394,000 grant from the Military Tri-Services Nursing Research program to study domestic violence. In 1996–99, the school received its first National Institutes of Health federal grants. Dr. Ann Newman's National Institutes of Nursing (NINR) grant built on her doctoral dissertation, which examined interventions to assist women in self-managing arthritis. Jane Neese, RN, PhD, established a grant built on her dissertation to study outcomes among elders using community-based programs. Peggy Wilmoth, RN, PhD, received a grant from the U.S. Department of Defense to study how enlisted women manage breast cancer while on active duty. These grants totaled over $1 million.

In 1998, the school had its first Distinguished Visiting Dean Colvard Professor, Laila Farhood, RN, PhD. She led a number of research seminars at the College of Nursing in 1998 and presented her research to the university. That year, the university appointed it first associate vice chancellor for Research.

By 2000, faculty members were applying for, and receiving, university and school grants to conduct research. They also successfully applied for Sigma Theta Tau research grants. For example, Linda Moore, RN, PhD, studied communication with individuals who had dementia. Dr. Peggy Wilmoth, RN, studied the psychosocial aspects of oncology. Dr. Linda Steele, RN, NP, studied women's health. And Sonya Hardin, RN, PhD, explored telehealth issues in nursing. In 2001, 13 faculty published articles in peer-reviewed journals or book chapters.

Dr. Debra Hymovich, RN, retired in the summer of 1999. In the fall, Dean Bishop hired William McAuley, PhD, as associate dean for Research beginning in January 2000.

Simultaneously, the College of Nursing hired its first endowed chair, Shirley Travis, RN, PhD, to continue her own program of research in the nursing care of aging populations and to mentor faculty. As part of the school's strategic plan, administrators recognized the need to reward faculty for research while offering programs to enhance research and scholarship skills. The school initiated a chapter of the National Gerontological Nursing Association. Its mission was to support research training for faculty by building partnerships between nurses and other disciplines and the community. In 2001, Dean Bishop hired Jackie Dienemann, RN, PhD, as a part-time research associate in the Office of Health Research to work directly with faculty across the college to support their research and scholarship.

In 2001, the College of Nursing received the A Sue Kerley Distinguished Nursing funding to pay for a leading nurse researcher to come to UNC Charlotte to mentor a research team and increase the visibility of nursing research across campus through a lecture. The first scholar was Dr. Barbara Holzclaw, RN; she did an assessment of research support needs in the school, presented a lecture, and led a research workshop. She also assisted in developing the call for proposals and plans to implement the faculty research section of the fund. In the spring of 2002, a call for proposals and a review resulted in formation of a research team, comprised of Leslie Hussey, RN, PhD, Sonya Hardin, RN, PhD, and Linda Steele, RN, PhD, that was chosen to study congestive heart failure.

In 2002–03, Ora Strickland, RN, PhD, became the second scholar. She mentored the Hussey/Hardin/Steele team, made a presentation to the university, and led a research workshop on women's health for the School of Nursing. The following year, Victoria Mock, RN, PhD, was named the third scholar. During her tenure, she assessed the research program, offered suggestions to enhance its productivity, mentored a research team, gave a lecture, and led a workshop.

In the fall of 2001, Dr. McAuley resigned, and the search began for a new associate dean for Research. The college continued to build infrastructure to support research. This also occurred at the university level. The school made arrangements to provide partial support for a biostatistician to assist faculty in proposal development and analysis after funding. In 2003, Dienemann was hired to be the chair of Adult Health and left the Office of Research. Dr. Travis departed the university leaving the Colvard Chair empty. That was also the first year that the faculty members' annual reviews included a category for scholarship as an expectation. In 2003, the college was reorganized with Dean Bishop, the new dean of the College of Health Professions. A reorganization added the Department of Public Health by recruiting new faculty and shifting Health Promotion faculty to the new department, then creating a School of Nursing. Pamala Larsen, RN, PhD, former associate dean for Academic Affairs, was made director of the School of Nursing. A committee was formed to develop a proposal for a PhD in the nursing program.

In 2006, the school's request for a doctoral program was denied, and the focus shifted to developing a DNP program and increasing its online offerings in graduate programs. The number of faculty has remained at 34, showing little growth from 32 in 1990. The Dean W. Colvard Endowed Chair is now a college professorship, and the school has a new endowment, the Carol Grotnes Belk endowed chair. There are now 18 faculty with doctorates and 16 with master's degrees. The culture of nursing research for all faculty has diminished but is hopefully on the rebound.

Two faculty members have been named Robert Wood Johnson Faculty Scholars, and one did postdoctoral training at UNC Chapel Hill. Five faculty members currently have strong programs of externally funded research: Donna Kazemi, RN,

PHD, prevention of substance abuse in college students; Christine Elnitsky, RN, PhD, community reintegration of veterans after deployment; Judith Cornelius, RN, PhD, prevention of HIV/AIDS in African American populations; Allison Burfield, RN, PhD, outcomes of mental health interventions; and Maren Coffman, RN, PhD, enhancement of self-management of diabetes in Latinas. Several others have well-developed programs of research nurtured through intramural and other grants. Thus, research and scholarship continue to be an integral part of the School of Nursing's mission. In the next 50 years, we hope to energize all faculty to more fully develop their research portfolios.

CHAPTER FIFTEEN

In Conclusion

Ann Mabe Newman

Whether you were a student in the 1960s, '70s, '80s, '90s, or 2000s, we hope you have seen yourself in these pages. We have changed the way we teach nursing over the past 50 years. Clinical and practice settings have changed. Uniforms have changed. Nurses are now expected to use evidence-based practices and conduct research. During the past two decades, we have embraced technology to enhance our teaching methods, our students' learning experiences, and their access to information.

Some of us don't realize how much technology and culture have changed in our lifetimes. Only 50 years ago:

- IV bottles were made of glass, and urinary catheters drained into glass bottles sitting on the floor.
- Nurses had to stand and give over their charts when a doctor entered the nurses' station.
- Bedpans were made of metal and were reusable.
- Wearing gloves was not a standard of care.
- Nurses smoked in the hospital and on the unit.
- Capping and pinning ceremonies were common but have now been replaced with white coat ceremonies.
- Dresses and white aprons have been exchanged for more modern white tops and pants for students; scrubs have replaced starched uniforms for nurses.
- Classes were all taught on campus. Now, many are taught online.
- Medications were dispensed in soufflé cups. Now, most medications come prepackaged.
- Patients used to request coffee, tea, and Coke. Now, they are likely to be served Frappuccino and smoothies as well.

- Paper charts have mostly switched to computer charting.
- HIPPA has changed the way nurses share information.
- Nurses now care for patients with diseases that were not known in the 1960s and '70s such as HIV/AIDS, SARS, and patients with heart, kidney, and other transplant surgeries, using the concept of infection control.
- Simulators were unheard of 50 years ago but are increasingly used to teach nursing students the skills they need in clinical practice.

Nursing has changed dramatically over the past 50 years. Nurses once gave baths and changed beds, did physical therapy, and dispensed medications. Now, nurses operate sophisticated machines and technology to assess and monitor their patients' health as well as planning patients' recovery, while still noticing subtle differences at the bedside and asking "what if" questions.

As we move forward over the next 50 years, nursing will continue to evolve but the basics won't change. We will always be our patients' advocates. We will continue to alleviate fear, relieve pain, use therapeutic touch, and practice evidence-based care. UNC Charlotte School of Nursing is dedicated to preparing students who want to enter the extraordinary world of nursing. There has never been a better time to be a nurse.

These two quotes summarize our charge:

Nursing is an art: and if it is to be made an art, it requires an exclusive devotion as hard a preparation as any painter's or sculptor's work; for what is the having to do with dead canvas or dead marble, compared with having to do with the living body, the temple of God's spirit? It is one of the Fine Arts: I had almost said, the finest of Fine Arts. — Florence Nightingale

Believe in nursing, in the wildest possible expanse of role and function, and believe so strongly that your beliefs can sustain you through the battles with the unknowing, unthinking, deluded, and barefoot pragmatists who wish to restrain the ideas and talents of nurses. — Donna Diers

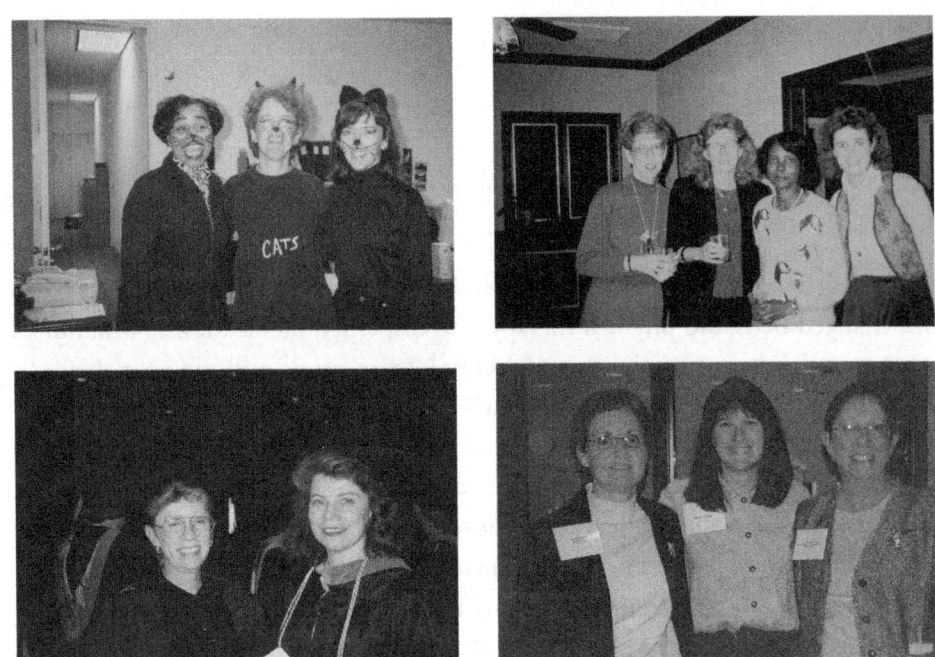

Faculty collage.

UNC Charlotte School of Nursing Alumni Chapter Distinguished Alumni

The School of Nursing and the School of Nursing Alumni Chapter (SONAC) host an annual Distinguished Alumni Lecture during which the Distinguished Nursing Alumni Award is presented. To date, seven individuals have received this award.

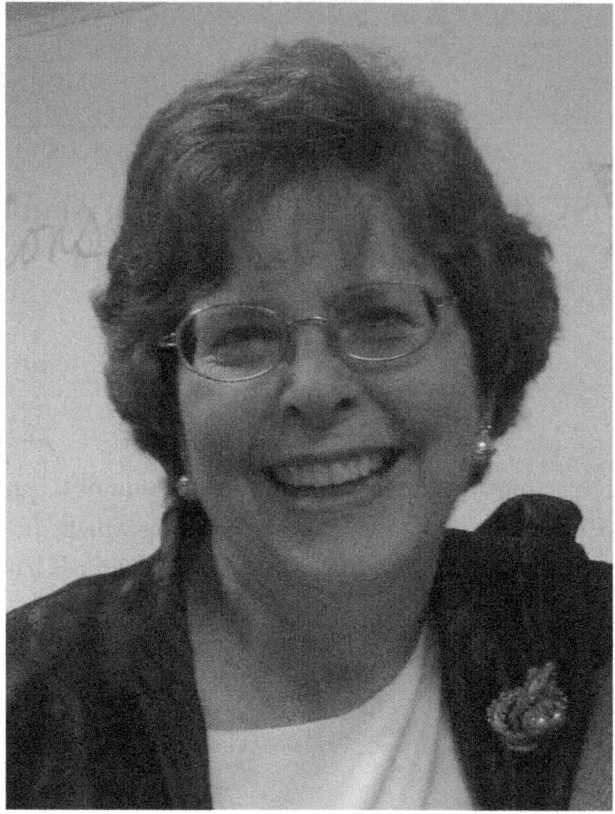

Lynda Opdyke.

2012 Distinguished Nursing Alumni: Lynda Opdyke

Lynda Opdyke Named First Distinguished Nursing Alumni[1]

Lynda Opdyke, MSN, RN, was named UNC Charlotte's 1st Distinguished Nursing Alumni by the University's School of Nursing Alumni Chapter. The announcement was made today by Dona Haney, Chapter President and Class of '69 '75 at the Chapter's inaugural event on Healthcare Reform: Implications for Health and Wellness held February 9th. The Distinguished Nursing Alumni award is bestowed upon an alum who has made outstanding contributions to the School of Nursing, and or recognized for exceptional achievement at the national, state or local levels.

Opdyke, who graduated in 1984, was in the first class that completed UNC Charlotte's MSN program. Classmates remember her as playing an instrumental role in advocating for the program. Letter-writing and ad campaigns were only a few strategies used by Opdyke and others to help bring a MSN program to UNC Charlotte.

Haney said: "Opdyke, throughout her career, has demonstrated extraordinary leadership in nursing education and is well deserving of this award." Opdyke, before her retirement in 2009, was the Associate Dean of Nursing at Mercy School of Nursing at Carolinas Medical Center. For 32 years at Mercy, Opdyke excelled as a nurse educator and advocate. Appointments included the NC Board of Nursing, National League for Nursing, and North Carolina Access to Health Care Task Force on Nursing.

Opdyke has presented over 70 presentations to professional, civic and faith groups on topics related to ethical decision-making, moral distress, child protection, test construction, program evaluation, end of life care and patient-centered care. Her awards are many, including two grants from the Duke Endowment for two studies on nurse retention, selection to The Great 100, recipient of the Pinnacle Award at Carolinas HealthCare System, and Sigma Theta Tau's Service Achievement award.

Since retirement, Opdyke continues to use her expertise of nursing education as she has been involved in supporting the development of the State Medical Assistance Team/ Medical Reserve Corp. She also volunteers as the Curator for the history museum at CMC-Mercy hospital. Opdyke is Ruling Elder at her church and has served or chaired committees on Child Protection, Stewardship, Worship and the Wedding Committee.

"Selection was difficult this year due to the many wonderful and outstanding nominees," says Baldwin, Associate Dean and Director of the School of Nursing. Baldwin said, "I am delighted that the School of Nursing Alumni Chapter decided to recognize its alums in this very special way. UNC Charlotte has a strong tradition of producing exceptional and high quality graduates who are making a difference in healthcare and improving the lives of others."

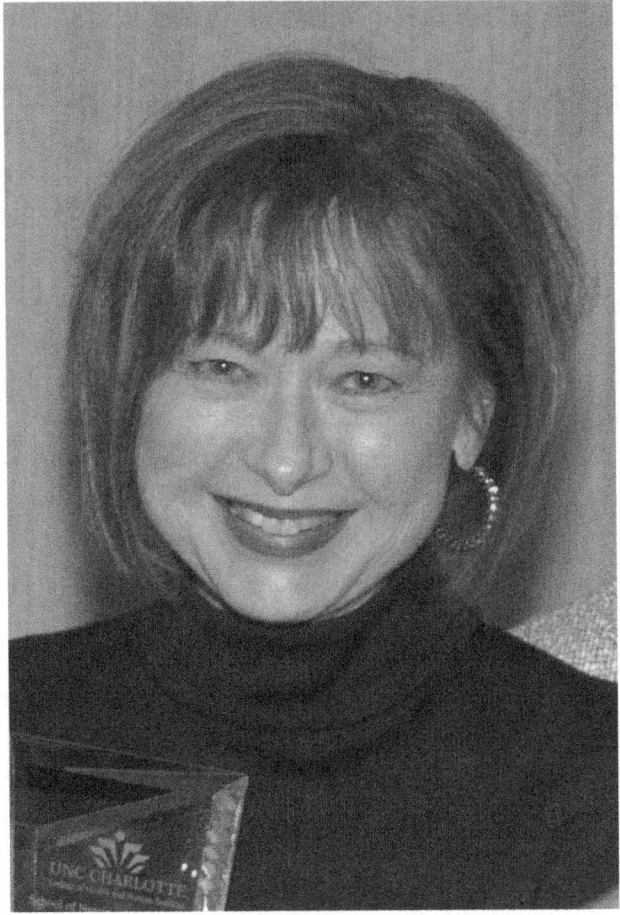

Dr. Pamela Rudisill.

2013 Distinguished Nursing Alumni: Dr. Pamela Rudisill
2013 Distinguished Alumni: Dr. Pamela Rudisill[2]

Pamela T. Rudisill was named UNC Charlotte's Distinguished Nursing Alumni by the University's School of Nursing Alumni Chapter.

The Distinguished Nursing Alumni Award is bestowed upon an alumnus or alumna who has made outstanding contributions to the School of Nursing or has been recognized for exceptional achievement at the national, state or local levels.

Rudisill, a graduate of the bachelor of science in nursing and master of science in nursing programs respectively, currently serves as Vice President and Chief Nursing Executive at Health Management Associates, Inc., where she heads up nursing/patient safety initiatives in the system's 71 hospitals. Among her many accomplishments at Health Management, she successfully implemented a Patient Safety Program to improve the care of the system's 1,560,000 yearly patients. She also served as Vice President of Nursing and Patient Safety during the four years prior to her 2012 executive appointment.

Rudisill began her career at Health Management as associate executive director and chief nursing officer in 1996, overseeing a $120 million budget for Nursing Services, Performance Improvement, Employee Health, Infection Control and Pharmacy at the system's Lake Norman Regional Medical Center in Mooresville.

She was appointed as an adjunct faculty member for UNC Charlotte's MSN program in 1990 and part-time professor of the same program in 2004.

"I think the Distinguished Nursing Alumni Award is a great way to recognize the wonderful contributions our alumni have made to healthcare and improving the lives of others," Dee Baldwin, Associate Dean and Director of the School of Nursing, said. "Our University has produced many exceptional graduates who have made major strides in the field of nursing."

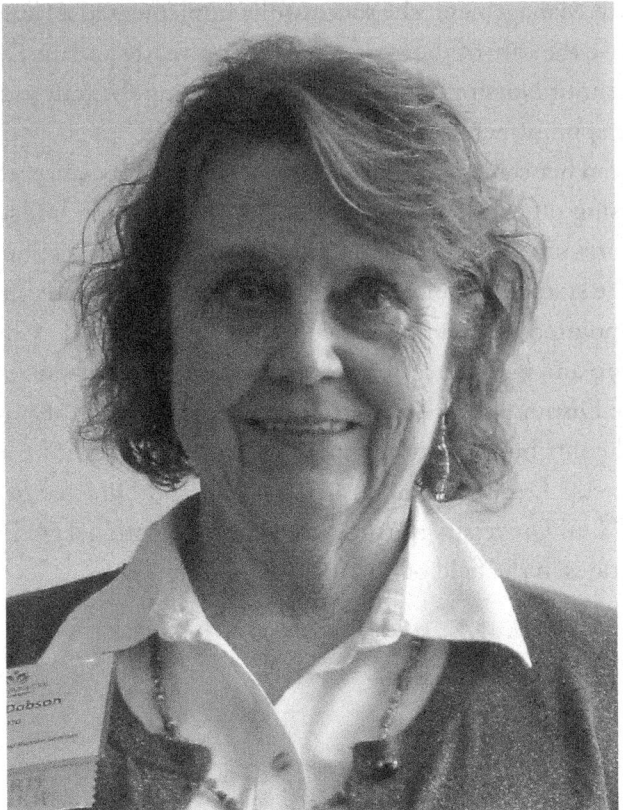

Lynn Dobson.

2014 Distinguished Nursing Alumni: Lynn Dobson
School of Nursing Names 2014 Distinguished Nursing Alumni[3]

UNC Charlotte School of Nursing Recognizes Distinguished Alumna for Outstanding Professional Service and Commitment to Improving the Lives of Others

The UNC Charlotte College of Health and Human Services' School of Nursing Alumni chapter recently honored Mrs. Lynn Dobson as the recipient of its 2014 Distinguished Alumni award. The award recognizes a UNC Charlotte nursing graduate for outstanding service to the School of Nursing or for recognition of exceptional achievement or state/national/international leadership in practical/clinical excellence, education, administration, research, or professional writing.

Dobson, a graduate of UNC Charlotte's Bachelor of Science in nursing and Master in Education programs, has dedicated more than three decades to the nursing profession. She is recognized as a passionate leader who has been a long-time advocate for children and vulnerable populations. Throughout her career, working in both North Carolina and South Carolina, Dobson has been involved in cancer care, Hospice, youth ministry, therapeutic child care programs, mission work and camps for special needs children.

"Lynn is an amazing person. A true humanitarian who exemplifies the spirit of the nursing profession," said Dr. Dee Baldwin, Associate Dean and Director of the School of Nursing. "She has not only made exceptional strides in the field but has made an indelible mark on communities both locally and globally. We are truly proud and honored to recognize her as one of our distinguished graduates."

Dobson has served as a Clinical Instructor in Pediatric Nursing at UNC Charlotte and is recognized as one of the three faculty members in the School of Nursing who led the effort to establish a nursing clinic for women and children at the Salvation Army. One of her major accomplishments in the Charlotte region was the development and direction of a summer program called Camp Care, which provides a camping opportunity for children with cancer. In 1992, she was honored with the Jefferson Award for her work with Camp Care. The Jefferson Award is given by WBTV and other community organizations given to individuals who enhance the community with their contributions.

Dobson was also instrumental in fund raising to deliver two ambulances to the Eleuthera (Bahamas) Emergency Preparedness Group and developing a seminar for cancer survivors on the island. Today, she continues to participate in Mission trips to the Bahamas and in 2010 received, along with her husband, the Outstanding Contribution to South Eleuthera Emergency Preparedness Organization award. She has also been honored by the Cancer Society of Eleuthera for her development of a seminar for cancer survivors.

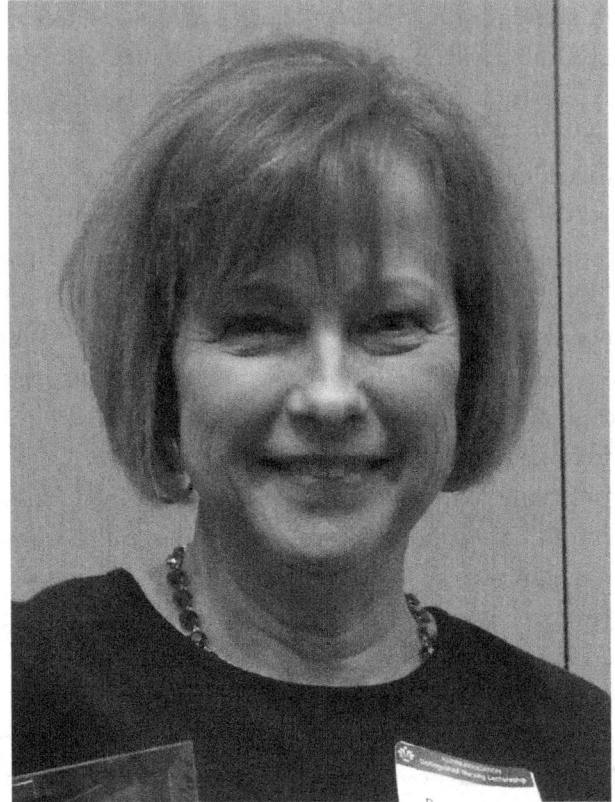

Pat Campbell.

2015 Distinguished Alumni: Pat Campbell
Pat Campbell Wins 4th Annual Distinguished Alumni Awards[4]

The School of Nursing has honored Patricia Campbell with its 4th Annual Distinguished Nursing Alumni Award.

Campbell, who received her undergraduate (84') and master's (88') nursing degrees from UNC Charlotte, is Vice President of Women's and Children's Services at Novant Health Charlotte.

Campbell has worked for Novant in women's and children's services since 1989, where she has been instrumental in the creation of many innovative initiatives, including a pediatric development program started in 2013.

CHHS Associate Dean and School of Nursing Director Dee Baldwin said though the selection this year was difficult, Campbell is a deserving candidate who continues a history of graduates making an impact.

"UNC Charlotte has a strong tradition of producing exceptional and high quality graduates who are making a difference in healthcare and improving the lives of others," Baldwin said.

During her tenure, Novant hospitals have been named the Best Place to Give Birth by *Charlotte Magazine,* a Friendly Business Work Place by the North Carolina Birthplace Coalition, and have been presented with the Snowmass Award for Women's Health.

Also a leader in the community, Campbell has served on the North Carolina Board of Nursing Directors and been a board member at local chapters of the March of Dimes and the Ronald McDonald House, among others.

She was named one of the 50 Most Influential Women by the *Mecklenburg Times* in 2012 and inducted into the American Academy of Nursing in 2013. Campbell is also the author of several books on critical care nursing.

She was honored at a ceremony at UNC Charlotte's Center City Campus earlier this semester.

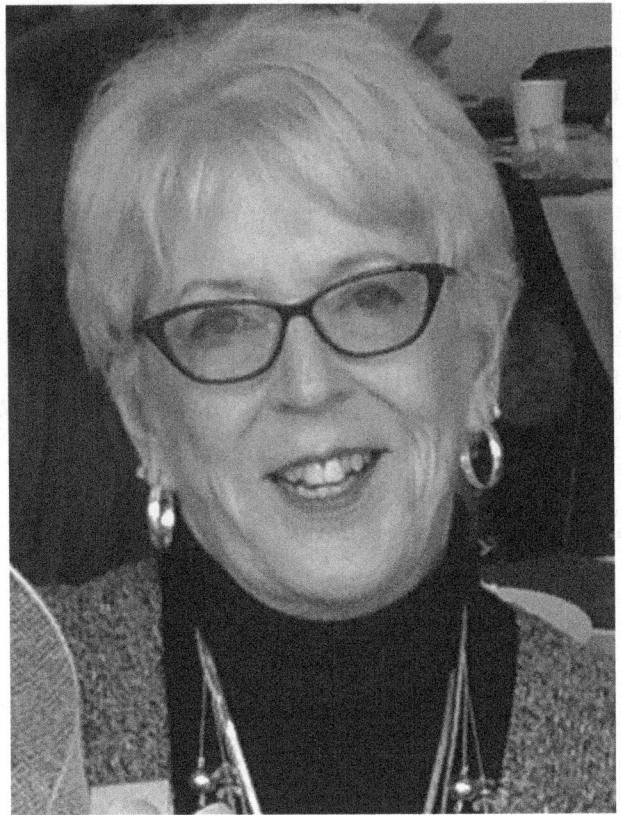

Dr. Ann M. Newman.

2016 Distinguished Nursing Alumni:
Ann Mabe Newman, RN, PhD
Ann M. Newman, 2016, Distinguished Alumni[5]

In 2016, Dr. Ann Mabe Newman, RN, PhD, was named as the Distinguished Nursing Alumni UNC Charlotte School of Nursing Alumni. In presenting the award, Dona Haney, RN, MSN, said there are few nursing alumni better known in the UNC system or the community. She went on to say: "Ann came to UNC Charlotte in 1971 to seek her BSN. She tells me her first day at UNC Charlotte was so frustrating she nearly did not return—but she did and she stayed. She is retired, but continues to consult."

Ann was an early student in our Pathways Program. She was a student representative on the planning team (she started her political activity early), upon graduation, she immediately entered our long-distance MSN program (which you will soon hear more about). She then started her educational career, and after a few years entered her doctoral program. (I am thinking she is one of our earliest alums to pursue a doctorate.)

Ann's career is filled with accolades and awards. If it is available to a nurse or a faculty member she has won it—Phi Beta Kappa, Sigma Theta Tau, Great 100, UNC Charlotte Hall of Fame, first recipient of the Elinor Brooks Caddell Faculty Scholar Award, UNC Charlotte's Nations Bank Teaching Excellence Award, and UNC Board of Governor's Award for Teaching Excellence (and I have summarized with a very short list).

Ann's career is one of service to nursing. Reading the list of who she has helped with theses and dissertations brings forth many familiar names. She is known as much for her community activity as she is for her educational activity. She has focused on psychiatric-mental health issues, arthritis, as well as cancer. Again, she received many accolades for her community work including being named "One of the 50 Most Influential Women in Charlotte" in 2010.

Ann promotes the concept that nurses are more knowledgeable of health care than anyone in the world. She is a supporter of nurses being involved in the political process, so much so that she ran a nearly successful campaign to become the first nurse in the N.C. House of Representatives in 2010. She actively protested the lack of Medicaid expansion in North Carolina. She was arrested (it was televised) and served 30 hours of community service (in which she helped the Arthritis Services write a grant). One of Ann's current American Nurses Association (ANA) projects is to get 10,000 nurses on boards by 2020, and she still signs her name Ann Newman, RN. I think you can see why our Selections Committee decided to add the title of UNC Charlotte School of Nursing Alumni Award to Ann Newman's CV.

At the UNC Charlotte Annual Alumni Awards Ceremony, on November 5, 2012, Dr. Ann Mabe Newman, RN ('78) was named to the University Hall of Fame.

Faculty Emerita Ann Mabe Newman Inducted into the University Hall of Fame[6]

A board-certified specialist in psychiatric nursing, Ann Mabe Newman has served as a practicing therapist in the community for more than 40 years. She retired from UNC Charlotte in July 2012 after three decades of teaching. During her tenure as an associate professor in the College of Health and Human Services School of Nursing, Newman taught courses on psychiatric-mental health nursing and health policy, and developed the university's online graduate program in Nursing Education.

Throughout her distinguished teaching and research career, Newman received numerous honors, including the prestigious Bank of American Award for Teaching Excellence. She also served on the N.C. State Board of Nursing and as president of the university's Faculty Council.

In the greater Charlotte community, Newman has served in volunteer positions with the PTA at Idlewild Elementary, Northeast Middle, and Independence High schools. She continues to provide pro bono healthcare services to the community, including grief and mental health counseling, advice on obtaining access to health services and information on how to manage chronic illnesses. In 2010, she was named one of the "50 Most Influential Women in Charlotte."

As a proud UNC Charlotte graduate ('78), Newman has undertaken a number of volunteer roles for the UNC Charlotte Alumni Association, including faculty advisor for the Nursing Alumni Interest Group, and member of the Alumni Association Board of Directors and the School of Nursing Alumni Chapter Board of Directors. She also was instrumental in establishing a nursing alumni emergency fund for UNC Charlotte SON students.

Newman received her diploma in Nursing from the University of Virginia before completing a Bachelor of Science degree in Nursing from UNC Charlotte in 1978. She went on to obtain a master's in Nursing from UNC Chapel Hill and a doctorate in nursing from the University of Alabama at Birmingham.

Through her devotion to teaching and service to UNC Charlotte and the greater community, Ann Mabe Newman has displayed the pioneering spirit of a 49er.

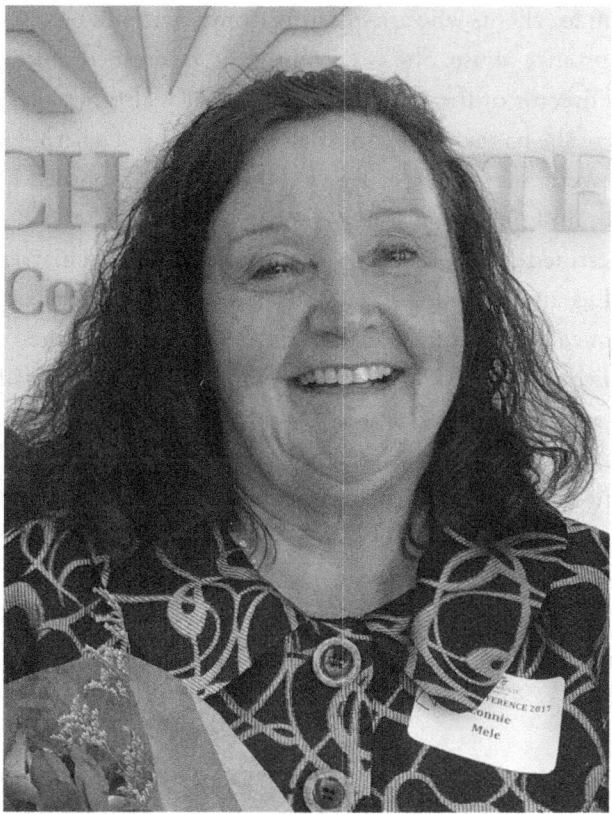

Connie Mele.

2017 Distinguished Nursing Alumni: Connie Mele, RN, MSN
Connie Mele '84 Named 6th Distinguished Nursing Alumni[7]

Connie Mele, MSN, RN, '84 has been named UNC Charlotte's 6th Distinguished Nursing Alumna by the School of Nursing alumni chapter. The Distinguished Nursing Alumni award is bestowed upon an alumni that has made outstanding contributions to the School of Nursing or been recognized for exceptional achievements in the field of nursing.

Mele is past President of the North Carolina Foundation Board for Alcohol and Drug Studies and Chair for the Addiction Nursing Certification Board. Under her leadership, the organization began the initial assessment to determine what was needed to accredit nurses who take this examination.

Mele was previously awarded a $1.5 million grant from SAMHSA (Substance Abuse, Mental Health Services Administration) to implement an integrated treatment program for clients who are suffering from severe and persistent mental illness as well as substance abuse. She is currently the Assistant Public Health Director and former Director of the Provided Behavioral Health Services of Mecklenburg County, where she has assisted with the development of a SAMHSA grant for Jail Diversion of Veterans who have PTSD (Post Traumatic Stress Disorder) or TBI (Traumatic Brain Injury).

Mele is certified as a Clinical Nurse Specialist in Psychiatric Mental Health Nursing and as an Advanced Practice Certified Addictions Nurse. She is also a Licensed Clinical Addiction Specialist and she is a board certified Nurse Executive.

As part of the class of 1984, Mele was among the first group of graduates from UNC Charlotte's MSN program.

"Selection for this distinguished honor remains difficult due to the many wonderful nominees," said Dee Baldwin, Associate Dean and Director of the School of Nursing. "I am delighted that the School of Nursing Alumni Chapter continues to recognize its alums in this very special way. UNC Charlotte has a strong tradition of producing high quality graduates who make a difference in the lives of others. Connie is one of those exceptional graduates."

NOTES

Introduction

1. "Proposed Curriculum," College of Nursing, UNC Charlotte, 1963, Nursing College 1965–88, UA0064, Boxes 1–4. J. Murrey Atkins Library, University of North Carolina at Charlotte.

2. UNC Charlotte School of Nursing, "Online Nursing Program Jumps in National Rankings," Charlotte, NC, Jan. 25, 2016, available at https://nursing.uncc.edu/news /2016–01–25/online-nursing-program-jumps-national-rankings.

3. UNC Charlotte, "School of Nursing Named a National Center of Excellence," *Inside UNC Charlotte,* Charlotte, NC, Oct. 18, 2016, available at https://inside.uncc.edu /news-features/2016–10–18/school-nursing-named-national-center-excellence.

4. Anonymous, "Bonnie Cone: Semi-retirement from a Growing Grandchild," *Carolina Journal* 9, no. 1 (July 3, 1973). Nursing College 1965–88, UA0064, Boxes 1–4. J. Murrey Atkins Library, University of North Carolina at Charlotte.

5. National League for Nursing, Washington, DC, 1963.

6. Bonnie Cone, "Application to Establish a School of Nursing," Charlotte, NC, 1964, College of Nursing, UNC Charlotte, 1963. Nursing College 1965–88, UA0064, Boxes 1–4. J. Murrey Atkins Library, University of North Carolina at Charlotte.

7. Anonymous, "N.C. Civitans Pick Bonnie as Best," Charlotte, NC, May 25, 1965, Nursing College 1965–88, UA0064, Boxes 1–4. J. Murrey Atkins Library, University of North Carolina at Charlotte.

8. Anonymous, "A Public Health President: Edith Brocker," *Tar Heel Nurse* 16 (December 1954).

9. Rosario A. Ortis, "Narrative Report for May 1953," Charlotte, NC, May 1953, Nursing College, 1965–88, UA0064, Boxes 1–4. J. Murrey Atkins Library, University of North Carolina at Charlotte.

10. Gerri Brady, in conversation with Dona Haney, April 2017.

11. Joyce Ann Lowder, personal account, Charlotte, NC, 2017. UNC Charlotte's College of Nursing unpublished archives.

12. Edith Brocker, "Factors for Consideration," Charlotte, NC, n.d., Nursing College 1965–88, UA0064, Boxes 1–4. J. Murrey Atkins Library, University of North Carolina at Charlotte.

13. Elinor Caddell, in conversation with Dona Haney, August 23, 2017.

14. Elinor Caddell, in conversation with Dona Haney, August 23, 2017.

15. Joyce Ann Lowder, personal account, Charlotte, NC, 2017. UNC Charlotte's College of Nursing unpublished archives.

16. Janet Kale Hunt, personal account, Charlotte, NC, 2017. UNC Charlotte's College of Nursing unpublished archives.

17. Dona Haney, personal account, Charlotte, NC, 2017. UNC Charlotte's College of Nursing unpublished archives.

18. Elinor Caddell, in conversation with Dona Haney, August 23, 2017.

19. Janet Kale Hunt, personal account, Charlotte, NC, 2017. UNC Charlotte's College of Nursing unpublished archives.

20. Gloria Johnson, personal account, Charlotte, NC, 2017. UNC Charlotte's College of Nursing unpublished archives.

21. Dona Haney, personal account, Charlotte, NC, 2017. UNC Charlotte's College of Nursing unpublished archives.

22. Janet Kale Hunt, personal account, Charlotte, NC, 2017. UNC Charlotte's College of Nursing unpublished archives.

23. Beth Donnelly, personal account, Charlotte, NC, 2017. UNC Charlotte's College of Nursing unpublished archives.

24. Janet Kale Hunt, personal account, Charlotte, NC, 2017. UNC Charlotte's College of Nursing unpublished archives.

25. Barbara Baker Mirgon, personal account, Charlotte, NC, 2017. UNC Charlotte's College of Nursing unpublished archives.

26. Shelia Frieze Nance, personal account, Charlotte, NC, 2017. UNC Charlotte's College of Nursing unpublished archives.

27. Dona Haney, personal account, Charlotte, NC, 2017. UNC Charlotte's College of Nursing unpublished archives.

1. The Beginning Years

1. Anonymous, "Nurse Training Program Activated," *The Charlotte Observer* (Charlotte, NC), Feb. 3, 1965. UNC Charlotte's College of Nursing unpublished archives.

2. Edith Brocker, "Annual Report," College of Nursing, UNC Charlotte, 1963, Nursing College 1965–88, UA0064, Boxes 1–4. J. Murrey Atkins Library, University of North Carolina at Charlotte.

3. Edith Brocker, "Annual Report," College of Nursing, UNC Charlotte, 1963, Nursing College 1965–88, UA0064, Boxes 1–4. J. Murrey Atkins Library, University of North Carolina at Charlotte.

4. Three-year diploma programs and two-year associate degree programs in nursing were the norm during this period of time, but only a four-year program was the goal of professional nursing. Diploma and associate degree programs entrance requirements were not as rigorous as those of baccalaureate programs.

5. Anonymous, "Nurse Training Program Activated," *The Charlotte Observer* (Charlotte, NC), Feb. 3, 1965. UNC Charlotte's College of Nursing unpublished archives.

6. Anonymous, "She's College Chairman of Infant Department," *The Charlotte*

Observer (Charlotte, NC), Jan. 30, 1966. UNC Charlotte's College of Nursing unpublished archives.

7. Edith Brocker, "First Annual Report of the Department of Nursing at UNC-C, September 1965–June 1966," College of Nursing, UNC Charlotte, 1966), Nursing College 1965–88, UA0064, Boxes 1–4. J. Murrey Atkins Library, University of North Carolina at Charlotte.

8. Anonymous, "Director Will Talk to Nurses," *Gastonia Gazette* (Gastonia, NC), Oct. 2, 1965.

9. Edith Brocker, "A Survey of Nursing Education Needs," Charlotte, NC, 1966.

10. "2nd Annual Report of the Department of Nursing, June 1, 1966 to May 31, 1967," College of Nursing, 1967, Nursing College 1965–88, UA0064, Boxes 1–4. J. Murrey Atkins Library, University of North Carolina at Charlotte.

11. "4th Annual Report of Activities of Nursing (June 1, 1968–May 31, 1969)," Charlotte, NC, 1969, Nursing College 1965–88, UA0064, Boxes 1–4. J. Murrey Atkins Library, University of North Carolina at Charlotte.

12. Tina Green, "Survey of Division of Nursing, University of North Carolina at Charlotte," Charlotte, NC, 1968, Nursing College 1965–88, UA0064, Boxes 1–4. J. Murrey Atkins Library, University of North Carolina at Charlotte.

13. D. W. Colvard, "The Chancellor's Report to the President for 1968–1969," UNC Charlotte, 1969. Personal collection of D. W. Colvard.

14. Elinor Caddell, in conversation with Dona Haney, Ann Newman, and Tina Wright, August 23, 2017. Nursing College 1965–88, UA0064, Boxes 1–4. J. Murrey Atkins Library, University of North Carolina at Charlotte.

15. D. W. Colvard, "A Named Professorship in Nursing," memo, Charlotte, NC, March 6, 1969, Nursing College 1965–88, UA0064, Boxes 1–4. J. Murrey Atkins Library, University of North Carolina at Charlotte.

16. This was a unique idea for 1969. It is what we now call social determinants of health and is being funded by the Robert Wood Johnson Foundation for a nationwide project called "Creating a Culture of Health."

17. A Nursing Clinic for Women and Children was developed in the 1990s by UNC Charlotte faculty and served as a clinical experience for students.

18. This important approach was the genesis for the creation of the College of Health and Human Services in which the School of Nursing is housed.

19. Geriatric Clinical Nurse Specialist and Geriatric Nurse Practitioner courses were offered in the School of Nursing.

20. This vision was realized in the 1980s when travel electives were developed.

21. Even though Dean Brocker did not have a doctorate, she understood the importance in academia.

22. Beth Donnelly, personal account, Charlotte, NC, 2017. UNC Charlotte's College of Nursing unpublished archives.

23. Dona Haney (class of '69) remembers the same patient fondly. She took care of him off and on for over six years.

24. Gloria Johnson, personal account, Charlotte, NC, 2017. UNC Charlotte's College of Nursing unpublished archives.

25. Susan Allen Henderson, personal account, Charlotte, NC, 2017. UNC Charlotte's College of Nursing unpublished archives.

26. Nancy Ann Kohler Rash, personal account, Charlotte, NC, 2017. UNC Charlotte's College of Nursing unpublished archives.

27. Janet Kale Hunt, personal account, Charlotte, NC, 2017. UNC Charlotte's College of Nursing unpublished archives.

28. Linda Turner, personal account, Charlotte, NC, 2017. UNC Charlotte's College of Nursing unpublished archives.

29. Dona Haney, personal account, Charlotte, NC, 2017. UNC Charlotte's College of Nursing unpublished archives.

30. Barbara Baker Mirgon, personal account, Charlotte, NC, 2017. UNC Charlotte's College of Nursing unpublished archives.

31. Kathleen Ledford Collins, personal account, Charlotte, NC, 2017. UNC Charlotte's College of Nursing unpublished archives.

32. Anonymous, "Kathleen Ledford Collins," obituary, Charlotte, NC, April 2013.

33. Kathleen Ledford Collins, personal account, Charlotte, NC, 2017. UNC Charlotte's College of Nursing unpublished archives.

34. Ruth Mauldin, personal account, Charlotte, NC, 2017. UNC Charlotte's College of Nursing unpublished archives.

35. Virginia Henderson, *The Principles and Practice of Nursing* (New York: Macmillan, 1978). UNC Charlotte's College of Nursing unpublished archives.

36. Joyce Ann Lowder, personal account, Charlotte, NC, 2017. UNC Charlotte's College of Nursing unpublished archives.

2. Rapid Growth and Development

1. Marinell Jernigan, "Annual Report (1972–1973)," UNC Charlotte College of Nursing, UNC Charlotte, 1973, Nursing College 1965–88, UA0064, Boxes 1–4. J. Murrey Atkins Library, University of North Carolina at Charlotte.

2. Marinell Jernigan, "Annual Report (1972–1973)," UNC Charlotte College of Nursing, UNC Charlotte, 1973, Nursing College 1965–88, UA0064, Boxes 1–4. J. Murrey Atkins Library, University of North Carolina at Charlotte.

3. UNC Charlotte, "1973–1974 University Catalog," UNC Charlotte, 1973–74, Nursing College 1965–88, UA0064, Boxes 1–4. J. Murrey Atkins Library, University of North Carolina at Charlotte.

4. Marinell Jernigan, "End-of-Course Report," UNC Charlotte College of Nursing, UNC Charlotte, 1973, Nursing College 1965–88, UA0064, Boxes 1–4. J. Murrey Atkins Library, University of North Carolina at Charlotte.

5. D. W. Colvard, letter, Charlotte, NC, 1974. UNC Charlotte's College of Nursing unpublished archives.

6. Newton Barnette, letter, Charlotte, NC, 1974. Personal collection of D. W. Colvard.

7. Bonnie Cone, letter, Charlotte, NC, 1974. Personal collection of D. W. Colvard.

8. Marinell Jernigan, "College of Nursing Annual Report of Dean Marinell Jernigan (to Chancellor)," Charlotte, NC, 1975), Nursing College 1965–88, UA0064, Boxes 1–4. J. Murrey Atkins Library, University of North Carolina at Charlotte.

9. Peggy Overcash, "Annual Report (1974–1975)," Charlotte, NC, 1975, Nursing College 1965–88, UA0064, Boxes 1–4. J. Murrey Atkins Library, University of North Carolina at Charlotte.

10. Marinell Jernigan, "College of Nursing Annual Report of Dean Marinell Jernigan (to Chancellor)," Charlotte, NC, 1975, Nursing College 1965–88, UA0064, Boxes 1–4. J. Murrey Atkins Library, University of North Carolina at Charlotte.

11. Marinell Jernigan, dean emerita, College of Nursing, UNC Charlotte, interview by Ann M. Newman, July 18, 2017.

12. Elinor Caddell, "Annual Report (1974)," College of Nursing, UNC Charlotte, 1974, Nursing College 1965–88, UA0064, Boxes 1–4. J. Murrey Atkins Library, University of North Carolina at Charlotte.

13. Ann Mabe Newman, personal account, Charlotte, NC, 2017. UNC Charlotte's College of Nursing unpublished archives.

14. Sally Reid Garrett, personal account, Charlotte, NC, 2017. UNC Charlotte's College of Nursing unpublished archives.

15. Lanny Ellis, personal account, Charlotte, NC, 2017. UNC Charlotte's College of Nursing unpublished archives.

16. Marilyn G. Smith, personal account, Charlotte, NC, 2017. UNC Charlotte's College of Nursing unpublished archives.

17. Lynn Dobson, personal account, Charlotte, NC, 2017. UNC Charlotte's College of Nursing unpublished archives.

18. Lucille Moses, personal account, Charlotte, NC, 2017. UNC Charlotte's College of Nursing unpublished archives.

19. Kathy Webb Barber, personal account, Charlotte, NC, 2017. UNC Charlotte's College of Nursing unpublished archives.

20. Janice Ellis, personal account, Charlotte, NC, 2017. UNC Charlotte's College of Nursing unpublished archives.

21. Sue Head, personal account, Charlotte, NC, 2017. UNC Charlotte's College of Nursing unpublished archives.

22. LaVerne Hicks Meyers, personal account, Charlotte, NC, 2017. UNC Charlotte's College of Nursing unpublished archives.

3. Conflict

1. Louise Schlachter, "College of Nursing Annual Report, June 3, 1982," Charlotte, NC, 1982, Nursing College 1965–88, UA0064, Boxes 1–4. J. Murrey Atkins Library, University of North Carolina at Charlotte.

2. Louise Schlachter, "College of Nursing Annual Report, June 3, 1982," Charlotte, NC, 1982, Nursing College 1965–88, UA0064, Boxes 1–4. J. Murrey Atkins Library, University of North Carolina at Charlotte.

3. Louise Schlachter, "Annual Report (1978–1979)," College of Nursing, UNC Charlotte, 1979.

4. Anonymous, personal account, Charlotte, NC, 1980.

5. Louise Schlachter, "Annual Report (1978–1979)," College of Nursing, UNC Charlotte, 1979, Nursing College 1965–88, UA0064, Boxes 1–4. J. Murrey Atkins Library, University of North Carolina at Charlotte.

6. Louise Schlachter, "Annual Report," Charlotte, NC, 1978, Nursing College 1965–88, UA0064, Boxes 1–4. J. Murrey Atkins Library, University of North Carolina at Charlotte.

7. Louise Schlachter, "1981–82 Annual Report College of Nursing (to Chancellor)," Charlotte, NC, 1982, Nursing College 1965–88, UA0064, Boxes 1–4. J. Murrey Atkins Library, University of North Carolina at Charlotte.

8. Ken Sanford, *Charlotte and UNC Charlotte: Growing Up Together* (Charlotte: University of North Carolina at Charlotte, 1996).

9. Louise Schlachter, "1981–82 Annual Report College of Nursing (to Chancellor)," Charlotte, NC, 1982, Nursing College 1965–88, UA0064, Boxes 1–4. J. Murrey Atkins Library, University of North Carolina at Charlotte.

10. Louise Schlachter, "1981–82 Annual Report College of Nursing (to Chancellor)," Charlotte, NC, 1982, Nursing College 1965–88, UA0064, Boxes 1–4. J. Murrey Atkins Library, University of North Carolina at Charlotte.

11. Sanford, *Charlotte and UNC Charlotte.*

4. A Year of Healing

1. Deeanna L. Burleson, personal account, Charlotte, NC, 2017. UNC Charlotte's College of Nursing unpublished archives.

2. Susan Hudson Marston, personal account, Charlotte, NC, 2017. UNC Charlotte's College of Nursing unpublished archives.

3. Nella Linker, personal account, Charlotte, NC, 2017. UNC Charlotte's College of Nursing unpublished archives.

4. Robyn Hill Turton, personal account, Charlotte, NC, 2017. UNC Charlotte's College of Nursing unpublished archives.

5. Lynda Colvard Opdyke, personal account, Charlotte, NC, 2017. UNC Charlotte's College of Nursing unpublished archives.

6. Datra Delk-Patrick, personal account, Charlotte, NC, 2017. UNC Charlotte's College of Nursing unpublished archives.

7. Teresa D. Parker, personal account, Charlotte, NC, 2017. UNC Charlotte's College of Nursing unpublished archives.

8. Delores Wong, personal account, Charlotte, NC, 2017. UNC Charlotte's College of Nursing unpublished archives.

9. Connie Mele, personal account, Charlotte, NC, 2017. UNC Charlotte's College of Nursing unpublished archives.

5. Regrouping, Moving Forward, Hitting Our Stride

1. Eileen A. Curran, personal account, Charlotte, NC, 2017. UNC Charlotte's College of Nursing unpublished archives.

2. Christian Carballo, personal account, Charlotte, NC, 2017. UNC Charlotte's College of Nursing unpublished archives.

6. Managing Change

1. Karen Schmaling, "Annual Report," College of Nursing, UNC Charlotte, 2006, Nursing College 1965–88, UA0064, Boxes 1–4. J. Murrey Atkins Library, University of North Carolina at Charlotte.

2. Karen Schmaling, "Annual Report," College of Nursing, UNC Charlotte, 2006, Nursing College 1965–88, UA0064, Boxes 1–4. J. Murrey Atkins Library, University of North Carolina at Charlotte.

3. Karen Schmaling, "Annual Report," College of Nursing, UNC Charlotte, 2006, Nursing College 1965–88, UA0064, Boxes 1–4. J. Murrey Atkins Library, University of North Carolina at Charlotte.

4. North Carolina State Board of Nursing, report, North Carolina State Board of Nursing, 1994, Nursing College 1965–88, UA0064, Boxes 1–4. J. Murrey Atkins Library, University of North Carolina at Charlotte.

5. JN Pease Architects, in conversation with Dean Bishop, 2000.

6. Yvonne Yousey, "A Night to Remember," personal account, Charlotte, NC, 2004. UNC Charlotte's College of Nursing unpublished archives.

7. Yvonne Yousey, "Update 2017," personal account, Charlotte, NC, 2017. UNC Charlotte's College of Nursing unpublished archives.

8. Tama Morris, "The School of Nursing and Hope," personal account, Charlotte, NC, 2004. UNC Charlotte's College of Nursing unpublished archives.

9. Bill Cody, "The Day Barbara Carper Hired Bill Cody at UNC Charlotte," personal account, Charlotte, NC, 2004. UNC Charlotte's College of Nursing unpublished archives.

10. Bill Cody, "Update Provided by Bill 9/17," personal account, Charlotte, NC, 2017. UNC Charlotte's College of Nursing unpublished archives.

11. Peggy Patton, "My Story," personal account, Charlotte, NC, 2004. UNC Charlotte's College of Nursing unpublished archives.

12. Meredith Flood, "Step by Step," personal account, Charlotte, NC, 2003. UNC Charlotte's College of Nursing unpublished archives.

13. Meredith Troutman-Jordan, "2017 Meredith Troutman Jordan," personal account, Charlotte, NC, 2017. UNC Charlotte's College of Nursing unpublished archives.

14. Lienne Edwards, "My Story," personal account, Charlotte, NC, 2004. UNC Charlotte's College of Nursing unpublished archives.

15. Diane Daniels, "A Good Beginning," personal account, Charlotte, NC, 2004. UNC Charlotte's College of Nursing unpublished archives.

16. Jackie Dienemann, "Candy," personal account, Charlotte, NC, 2004. UNC Charlotte's College of Nursing unpublished archives.

7. Into a New Century, Implications/Adjustments to a New Structure

1. Karen Schmaling, "Annual Report," College of Nursing, UNC Charlotte, 2008, Nursing College 1965–88, UA0064, Boxes 1–4. J. Murrey Atkins Library, University of North Carolina at Charlotte.

2. Karen Schmaling, "Annual Report," College of Nursing, UNC Charlotte, 2006, Nursing College 1965–88, UA0064, Boxes 1–4. J. Murrey Atkins Library, University of North Carolina at Charlotte.

3. Karen Schmaling, "Executive Summary of Annual Progress in Achieving 2005–2010 Strategic Plan Goals," College of Nursing, UNC Charlotte, 2010, Nursing College 1965–88, UA0064, Boxes 1–4. J. Murrey Atkins Library, University of North Carolina at Charlotte.

4. Karen Schmaling, "Annual Report," College of Nursing, UNC Charlotte, 2007, Nursing College 1965–88, UA0064, Boxes 1–4. J. Murrey Atkins Library, University of North Carolina at Charlotte.

10. Recognition, Successes, New Programs in Nursing

1. UNC Charlotte School of Nursing, "Online Nursing Program Jumps in National Rankings," Charlotte, NC, Jan. 25, 2016, available at https://nursing.uncc.edu/news/2016–01–25/online-nursing-program-jumps-national-rankings.

2. Aly Bell, personal account, Charlotte, NC, 2017. UNC Charlotte's College of Nursing unpublished archives.

3. Janis Joyce, personal account, Charlotte, NC, 2017. UNC Charlotte's College of Nursing unpublished archives.

4. Jackie Dienemann, personal account, Charlotte, NC, 2017. UNC Charlotte's College of Nursing unpublished archives.

11. Beyond the Classroom

1. A note indicates that the award now includes a monetary award.

2. Betsy McLean, "New Award Creating Tradition," *New Notes* (Charlotte, NC), n.d. From UNC Charlotte's College of Nursing unpublished archives.

3. Dee Baldwin, in discussion with Dona Haney, Nov. 9, 2017.

4. Dee Baldwin, in discussion with Dona Haney, Nov. 9, 2017.

5. Gamma Iota, "STTI Organizational Fact Sheet," *Chapter Archives, Sigma Theta Tau International,* Nov. 6, 2017, available at www.sigmanursing.org.

6. Gamma Iota, "STTI Organizational Fact Sheet," *Chapter Archives, Sigma Theta Tau International,* Nov. 6, 2017, available at www.sigmanursing.org.

7. Gamma Iota, "STTI Organizational Fact Sheet," *Chapter Archives, Sigma Theta Tau International,* 2017, Nov. 6, 2017, available at www.sigmanursing.org.

8. Gamma Iota, "STTI Organizational Fact Sheet," *Chapter Archives, Sigma Theta Tau International,* Nov. 6, 2017, available at www.sigmanursing.org.

9. Polly Paddock, "Homeless Women Get Nurse Care," *The Charlotte Observer* (Charlotte, NC), May 5, 1991, Nursing College 1965–88, UA0064, Boxes 1–4. J. Murrey Atkins Library, University of North Carolina at Charlotte.

10. Polly Paddock, "Homeless Women Get Nurse Care."

11. Polly Paddock, "Homeless Women Get Nurse Care."

12. Endowed Scholarships and Funds

1. University Advancement, "Endowed Scholarships and Funds," UNC Charlotte, n.d. UNC Charlotte's College of Health and Human Services archives.

13. Named Areas within the College of Nursing

1. College of Health and Human Services, "Named Areas within the College of Nursing" (report, UNC Charlotte, n.d.). UNC Charlotte's College of Health and Human Services archives.

Appendix

1. UNC Charlotte School of Nursing, "Lynda Opdyke Named First Distinguished Nursing Alumni," Charlotte, NC, 2012, https://nursing.uncc.edu/news/2012–02–27/linda-opdyke-named-first-distinguised-nursing-alumni.

2. UNC Charlotte School of Nursing, "2013 Distinguished Alumni: Dr. Pamela Rudisill," Charlotte, NC, 2013, https://nursing.uncc.edu/news/2013–02–12/2013-distinguished-alumni-dr-pamela-rudisill.

3. UNC Charlotte School of Nursing, "School of Nursing Names 2014 Distinguished Nursing Alumni," Charlotte, NC, 2014, https://nursing.uncc.edu/news/2014–03–25/school-nursing-names-2014-distinguished-nursing-alumni.

4. UNC Charlotte School of Nursing, "Pat Campbell Wins 4th Annual Distinguished Alumni Award," Charlotte, NC, 2015, https://nursing.uncc.edu/news/2015–04–09/pat-campbell-wins-4th-annual-distinguished-alumni-award.

5. Dona Haney, "Ann M. Newman, 2016, Distinguished Alumni," Charlotte, NC, Feb. 9, 2016).

6. UNC Charlotte School of Nursing, "Faculty Emeritus Ann Mabe Newman Inducted into the University Hall of Fame," Charlotte, NC, 2012, https://nursing.uncc.edu news/2012–11–05/faculty-emeritus-ann-mabe-newman-inducted-university-hall-fame.

7. UNC Charlotte School of Nursing, "Connie Mele '84 Named 6th Distinguished Nursing Alumni," Charlotte, NC, 2017, https://nursing.uncc.edu/news/2017–03–15 /connie-mele'84-named-6th-distinguished-nursing-alumni.

INDEX

Page numbers in italics refer to illustrations.

Made in United States
Orlando, FL
22 March 2026

79568417R00138